CASCADIA SCORECARD 2006

OTHER SIGHTLINE INSTITUTE TITLES

Cascadia Scorecard 2005:
Focus on Energy

Cascadia Scorecard:
Seven Key Trends Shaping the Northwest

This Place on Earth 2002:
Measuring What Matters

This Place on Earth 2001:
Guide to a Sustainable Northwest

State of the Northwest, revised 2000 edition

Seven Wonders

Green-Collar Jobs

Tax Shift

Over Our Heads:
A Local Look at Global Climate

Misplaced Blame:
The Real Roots of Population Growth

Stuff: The Secret Lives of Everyday Things

This Place on Earth:
Home and the Practice of Permanence

The Car and the City

Hazardous Handouts

State of the Northwest

CASCADIA SCORECARD

SEVEN KEY TRENDS SHAPING THE NORTHWEST

2006

FOCUS ON SPRAWL & HEALTH

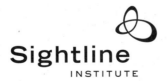

Sightline
INSTITUTE

SIGHTLINE INSTITUTE (formerly Northwest Environment Watch)
is a not-for-profit research and communication center in Seattle, Washington.
Its mission is to promote a sustainable economy and way of life throughout
the Pacific Northwest—the biological region stretching from southeast Alaska
to northern California and from the Pacific Ocean to the crest of the Rockies.

Library of Congress Control Number: 2006903211
ISBN 1-886093-16-4
(ISBN-13: 978-1-886093-16-4)

Design, production, and illustration: Jennifer Shontz
Editing: Julie Van Pelt
Proofreading: Sherri Schultz

Printed by Transcontinental Printing, Canada, with vegetable-based ink on
recycled paper. Text: 100 percent postconsumer waste, bleached without
chlorine; map pages: 10 percent postconsumer, bleached without chlorine.

Sightline Institute is a 501(c)(3) tax-exempt organization. To order
publications, become a member, or learn more, please contact:

SIGHTLINE INSTITUTE
1402 Third Avenue, Suite 500
Seattle, WA 98101-2130 USA
(206) 447-1880; fax (206) 447-2270
www.sightline.org

CONTENTS

CASCADIA AND
ITS SCORECARD

This book begins with place: Cascadia, the Pacific Northwest. Encompassing most of British Columbia, Idaho, Washington, Oregon, and adjoining parts of Alaska, Montana, and California (see map inside front cover), Cascadia is a region with a dawning sense of itself. Its population is larger than that of the Netherlands, its economy is larger than Russia's, and its land area is larger than France, Germany, and the United Kingdom combined—with Belgium, Italy, and Switzerland thrown in for good measure.

Named for the Cascade Mountains, the earthquake-prone Cascadia subduction zone offshore under the Pacific, and—above all—for the cascading waterfalls that pepper the region, Cascadia has a common indigenous cultural heritage and a common history. It is bound by salmon and rivers, snowcapped mountains and towering forests. Its people share not only geography but also an aspiration: to live well in their place.

Cascadia has traditions of innovation in the public and private sectors, a well-educated populace, and a long-standing commitment to conservation and quality of life. These traits show: the Northwest retains a larger share of its natural heritage intact than perhaps any other part of the industrial world and has helped set the conservation agenda for the continent.

Still, Cascadians are in only the early phases of rising to the next great challenge for humanity: gradually but fundamentally realigning the human enterprise so that both the economy and its supporting ecosystems can thrive. Daunting, complex, systemic, seemingly quixotic, this goal—

balancing people and place—is nonetheless more attainable here than anywhere else on this continent. If northwesterners can reconcile themselves with their landscapes, they can set an example for the world.

The Cascadia Scorecard, a project started in 2004 by Sightline Institute (formerly Northwest Environment Watch), measures long-term progress in the Pacific Northwest. An index of seven trends shaping the future of the region, it is a simple but surprisingly far-reaching gauge. The Scorecard's indicators—health, economy, population, energy, sprawl, wildlife, and pollution—provide status reports for Cascadia and, by highlighting successful communities, offer a practical vision for a better Northwest.

If northwesterners can reconcile themselves with their landscapes, they can set an example for the world

Above all, the Scorecard puts a spotlight on the long view and the questions that most matter over great spans of time: Are we living longer, healthier lives? Are we building strong human communities? Are we handing down to our children a place whose economy is fair and whose natural heritage is regenerating?

This 2006 edition of the Cascadia Scorecard is the third book in a series. The first book, *Cascadia Scorecard 2004*, presented a complete exposition of the seven trends: why they matter, what they mean, and what Cascadians can do about them. The second book, *Cascadia Scorecard 2005*, updated the Scorecard and focused on the one trend—energy—on which the region most lags behind world leaders. *Cascadia Scorecard 2006* does not aspire to replace previous editions in the series; it is an update and companion to the previous books.

Cascadians who wish to learn more about the Scorecard and how to turn its indicators in the right direction can find and download ample additional information—including maps and charts in a number of formats, supplementary state-, provincial-, and local-level Scorecard data, and a version of this book with complete sources and citations—at *www. sightline.org*. While there, they can sign up for free electronic updates of the Scorecard by subscribing to one of our several email newsletters.

Where are the citations?

A footnoted and annotated online version of *Cascadia Scorecard 2006* is posted at *www.sightline.org*. It contains notes with full documentation in support of factual statements in this book, along with animated, time-lapse versions of many Scorecard maps. It also offers supplementary data, technical material, links, and notes on methods and definitions.

INTRODUCTION: VITAL SIGNS

Unforeseen, and perhaps unforeseeable, events dominated Cascadia's headlines in 2005 and early 2006. Two flukes of weather half a continent away—Hurricanes Katrina and Rita—drove up gasoline prices and drained tens of millions of dollars from the Northwest economy. Health departments braced themselves for outbreaks of avian flu. Unexpectedly sharp increases in the cost of medical care fueled debates over cutbacks (in British Columbia) and expansions (in Oregon) in public health. And a near-total failure of salmon runs in southern Oregon and northern California led to an unprecedented closure of that region's commercial fishery.

If these disparate events have a unifying theme, it is that complicated systems—economies, ecosystems, and bodies alike—can be more fragile than they seem. Most of the time they function smoothly and predictably. But when an unforeseen shock sends them out of balance—as at the onset of illness, recession, or species collapse—their behavior all too often seems governed by chance rather than fixed laws.

Undaunted or even spurred on by such mysteries, legions of specialists dedicate their lives to understanding the systems that most affect us: measuring their condition, tallying their inputs and outputs, and identifying the leverage points—simple interventions, really—that can do the most good for our health, our livelihoods, and our natural heritage. In a sense, then, Cascadia's medical researchers, economists, and biologists are all engaged in the same kind of work: understanding and improving the health of our place.

Like a healthy body, a healthy place is resilient, able to heal itself. It can absorb stresses and shocks—an unexpected economic jolt, a bout of bad weather—and it anticipates hazards without overreacting. Measuring the health of a place requires a variety of tools and approaches; a single gauge can't capture it.

But our government and society still tend to reckon collective well-being in one common unit: dollars. Just as the robustness of an economy is commonly gauged by the dollar value of total output—as measured by gross domestic product, or GDP—policy makers and pundits alike seem ever more inclined to view health, both human and wild, through the lens of our finances. For example, the rising cost of medical care—and who pays for it—dominates the political debate over human health. Similarly, press accounts all too frequently portray the preservation of native landscapes as financial sacrifices rather than as expressions of responsible stewardship of our shared inheritance.

Better measures of progress are essential to achieving a fuller tally of the region's well-being

A steely-eyed financial accounting of Cascadia's health does have its place. But undue attention to the bottom line focuses our attention on the costs of achieving progress rather than on the benefits of realizing our shared aspirations. As important, an excessive focus on monetary costs blinkers our outlook by drawing our thoughts to the most expensive symptoms—burgeoning medical bills, for example—rather than leading us to the simplest and most cost-effective cures.

Better measures of progress—measures that recognize our shared desire for strong and healthy human communities and thriving natural ones—are essential to achieving a fuller tally of the region's well-being. The Cascadia Scorecard is designed with this in mind. A simple yet broad-ranging yardstick, the Scorecard tracks long-term progress toward creating a healthy, lasting prosperity grounded in place.

The 2006 edition of the Cascadia Scorecard takes health, not just of people but of place, as its theme and organizing principle. And it includes a special section on how improvements on one Scorecard trend—sprawl—can yield surprising health benefits.

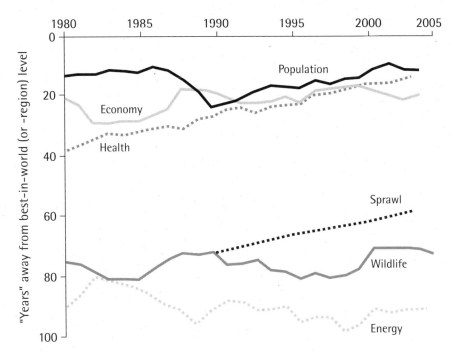

Figure 1.
Human impacts
on nature score
substantially worse
than indicators of
human well-being.

Overall, *Cascadia Scorecard 2006* reveals a place whose human inhabitants are faring comparatively well. The exceptions are notable— the region struggles with entrenched poverty and searing economic and social inequities. Still, the Scorecard indicators show that Cascadians are generally healthy and wealthy, and—in their childbearing—increasingly wise. By the Scorecard's reckoning, Cascadia notches its best performance in health, economy, and population (see Figure 1).

But our way of life is placing unprecedented strains on nature. The iconic wildlife of our place—salmon, orcas, and wolves among them—are far less abundant than they once were. And our lifestyles, particularly our consumption of energy and the sprawl of our cities, are placing new stresses on our climate and threatening the integrity of our remaining wild places. The indicators of sprawl, wildlife populations, and especially energy are the farthest from the Scorecard's goals.

Over the course of two and a half decades, the region's aggregate score on the Scorecard has slowly climbed, buoyed primarily by steady gains in health and a gradual improvement, at least since the mid-1980s, in the design of our cities (see Figure 2). But compared with models from around the world—Japan for health, Germany for energy, and so on—Cascadia lags an average of 44 years behind (see Table 1). That is, based on the Scorecard's reckoning, it would take 44 years of slow-and-steady progress to bring Cascadia's performance up to what those places had already achieved in 2001 or 2002. Meanwhile, the regions in the world that perform best on these indicators are not standing still but are racking up further improvements. Life expectancy in Japan, for example, has increased by nearly a year since the Cascadia Scorecard was introduced in 2004.

Progress on the Scorecard trends was by far quickest from the late 1990s through 2001, which was a time of broadly shared gains in economic prosperity and a period of increases in the populations of several sentinel species, particularly wolves and salmon. But since the new millennium, the rate of increase has resumed the slower pace characteristic of the 1980s. Indeed, from 2001 through 2003, the aggregate value of the Cascadia Scorecard barely budged. It ticked up only slightly in 2004. Preliminary figures for 2005 suggest that the Scorecard likely experienced a modest rise.

The seven Scorecard trends have never moved in lockstep. In the most recent year for which data are available, for example, the Scorecard's human health, economy, energy, and sprawl indicators made modest improvements. But those advances were partially counterbalanced by declines in key wildlife populations.

Three notes of caution are in order. First, any aggregation of such disparate trends can never be definitive; it can only be indicative, as detailed in previous editions of *Cascadia Scorecard*. Second, the wildlife indicator is a new addition to the Scorecard; it takes the place of the forest indicator of the previous two editions, which was based on analysis

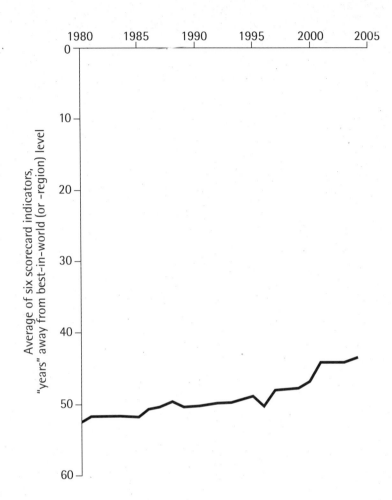

Figure 2.
Progress on the
Scorecard's indicators
has stalled after
steady improvement
in the 1990s.

of data from a satellite system that is now malfunctioning. This change
required recalibrating the Cascadia Scorecard from previous years.

Third, detailed time-series trends for the Scorecard's pollution indicator are not yet available and therefore are not included in the aggregate
score for the Scorecard. We do know that regional levels of toxic flame
retardants, or PBDEs—one of several pollutants that the Scorecard
tracks—have grown alarmingly over the past several decades. Levels
in northwesterners' bodies appear to be at least 20 times higher today

Key trend	Indicator	Target: Place with excellent—and achievable—record	Target
Health	Life expectancy at birth, in years	Japan, 2001	81.3 years
Economy	Composite index of unemployment rate, median income, and poverty rate, 1990 = 100	Selected high-performing states, provinces, and European nations, recent years	108.6 points
Population	Total fertility rate, in children born per woman	Netherlands and Sweden, 2001–02	1.7 births
Energy	Per capita use of highway fuel and nonindustrial electricity, in gallons of gasoline-equivalent per week	Germany, 2001	7.4 gallons
Sprawl	Percentage of metropolitan-area residents in compact, transit-friendly neighborhoods	Interim target: Vancouver, BC, 2001 (European and wealthy Asian cities do better, but data not comparable.)	62 percent
Wildlife	Populations of five key "indicator species," as a percentage of historic abundance	Interim target: between one-third and one-half of levels prior to European colonization, depending on the species	43 percent
Pollution	Median concentration of toxic chemicals in breastmilk, in parts per billion	PBDEs: median levels in Japan, 2000 PCBs: lowest level found in Sightline study, samples collected in 2003	1.3 parts per billion PBDEs, 49 parts per billion PCBs
Average:			

Table 1. Cascadia Scorecard 2006: The Northwest will require some 44 years of steady progress to meet ambitious, but achievable, goals.

Cascadia Scorecard 2006	Scorecard gap With steady progress, how many years to match target?	Status and trend
79.4 years	12 years	Eighth best in world; improving slowly.
100.3 points	20 years	Strong by international standards; underperforming national averages since 1990; improved in 2004.
1.81 births	11 years	Close to world's best, but variable; substantial progress since 1990, but worsened slightly in 2003 and 2004.
14.5 gallons	91 years	Worst performance among Scorecard trends; improved since 1999, but no net progress over 25 years.
33 percent	57 years	Steady but modest improvements in recent years; region still lags far behind Vancouver, BC.
15 percent	71 years	Variable, with recent improvements in wolf populations partially offset by declines in caribou.
50 parts per billion, PBDEs; 134 parts per billion, PCBs	? years (Time-series data unavailable.)	PBDEs among highest in world, concentrations likely rising; PCB levels apparently lower than national averages from previous decades, though precise comparisons are difficult.
	44 years	Improved fastest in late 1990s; slow improvements in the new millennium.

than in the mid-1980s. However, some evidence suggests that levels of a related class of toxic contaminants, PCBs, are no longer increasing and may even be slowly declining.

Shifting Scorecard trends to a healthier trajectory will require more than a clear-eyed diagnosis of the region's condition. It will also require effective prescriptions for change. Especially effective are modest shifts in Cascadians' policies and behaviors that can improve several Scorecard trends at the same time. Such systemic innovations—which we cover in the book's conclusion—are already emerging. Indeed, they have been gathering momentum for some time, proving their potential and, often, their profitability. All that is lacking is a critical mass of northwesterners acting in their own lives and through the region's governments, businesses, and civic organizations to speed the change.

1. ECONOMY

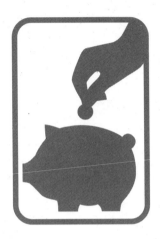

Sheer bulk reveals no more about the health of an economy than about the health of a person. Yet the most-used economic indicator is gross domestic product (GDP), which reflects sheer economic bulk—total sales of finished goods and services. In Cascadia, GDP growth is a poor indicator, at best, for how the economy is working for ordinary people. The Scorecard's four-part measure of economic security—combining data on unemployment, poverty, child poverty, and median income—reveals that many middle- and lower-income residents of the Northwest states face precarious economic conditions.

As of 2004, Sightline's economic security indicator for the Northwest states had made only minuscule gains compared with 1990, the reference year for Scorecard trends (see Figure 3). And the region's performance has lagged behind the rest of the nation. Over the 14-year period from 1990 to 2004, Washington was one of only two states (along with Hawaii) to show no net improvement in its economic security indicator. Oregon's improvement was vanishingly small, tied for 48th place among the 50 states.

Meanwhile, many other states posted substantial progress in reducing poverty and boosting incomes and employment. At the beginning of the 1990s Washington ranked 12th best among US states on the Scorecard's economic security indicator, while Oregon ranked 22nd. By 2004 the states had sunk to 27th and 34th place, respectively. Idaho did somewhat better, ending the period at nearly the same rank at which it had begun.

Washington's stagnation can be attributed to a poverty rate that grew from less than 10 percent—one of the lowest in the nation in the early 1990s—to nearly 12 percent in recent years. Unemployment

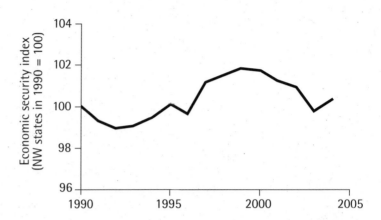

Figure 3.
The Northwest
states have posted
minimal gains in
economic security
since 1990.

also climbed in the Evergreen State. Oregon's poor showing is the result of ballooning unemployment—the highest in the nation between 2002 and 2004—and stagnating income. By 2004, Oregon's median household income (adjusted for inflation) had returned nearly to its 1990 level, while national median income rose by more than $2,000 during the period. In contrast, Idaho saw broad improvement across every measure of economic security. Idaho's rates of poverty and child poverty have declined since 1990, as did the unemployment rate. And middle-class residents of the state prospered, as median household income rose by $5,700 (after adjusting for inflation).

The good news for the Northwest is that unemployment rates are already declining, perhaps a sign of a brighter economic future for lower- and middle-income residents. To help ordinary families achieve economic security, and to regain their once-enviable ranks among the states, Oregon and Washington will need to boost median wages and pursue measures to reduce poverty and child poverty.

British Columbia registered a small increase in economic security in 2003, the most recent year with full data available, after suffering declines in the two years prior (see Figure 4). Small reductions in the share of all residents and children below the low-income cutoff (sometimes referred to as Canada's poverty rate), as well as in the unemployment rate, were responsible for British Columbia's uptick. Unfortunately, in inflation-adjusted terms, the province's median income declined slightly, continuing a trend that began in 2000. And British Columbia continues to lag behind the rest of Canada—and even behind its own performance in the early 1990s.

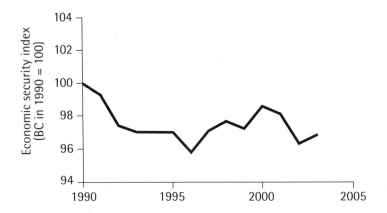

Figure 4. British Columbia's economic security is still below its 1990 level, largely due to a fall in median income.

2. POPULATION

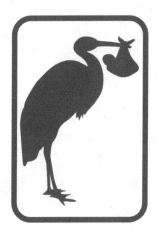

Cascadia's slow-motion revolution in reproduction—the shift toward smaller families, later in life—continued in 2004, the last complete year for which data are available. Average family size remained roughly stable at 1.8 children (see Figure 5).

Average family size (lifetime births per woman or, more precisely, the "total fertility rate") is an excellent gauge of well-being for women and families. It tends to decline when opportunities open to women, when child poverty and sexual abuse diminish, and when contraceptive availability improves. Family size is also a gauge of the Northwest's population growth, which powerfully shapes the region's environment. Births—unlike migration—account for the share of this population growth that is most clearly under the control of the region's residents. Finally, trends in family size deeply influence the housing market and resulting construction patterns.

Decreasing births among young women contributed to the region's overall 2004 stability in family size. For the second year running, Cascadia's teen birthrate was at a record low, with just under 27 births per 1,000 teenage girls in the region. Births among women in their early 20s declined as well. In British Columbia, births to thirtysomethings overtook births to twentysomethings in 2004—an unprecedented fertility pattern in Cascadia (see Figure 6).

Progress toward smaller, later families is also shaping the composition of households. The share of Cascadian households that have no children in them is steadily expanding, reaching 68 percent in 2000. Childless younger and older adults, who are more likely to welcome apartment or condominium dwellings than families with children, are a growing share of the housing market. Cascadia's share of single-person households,

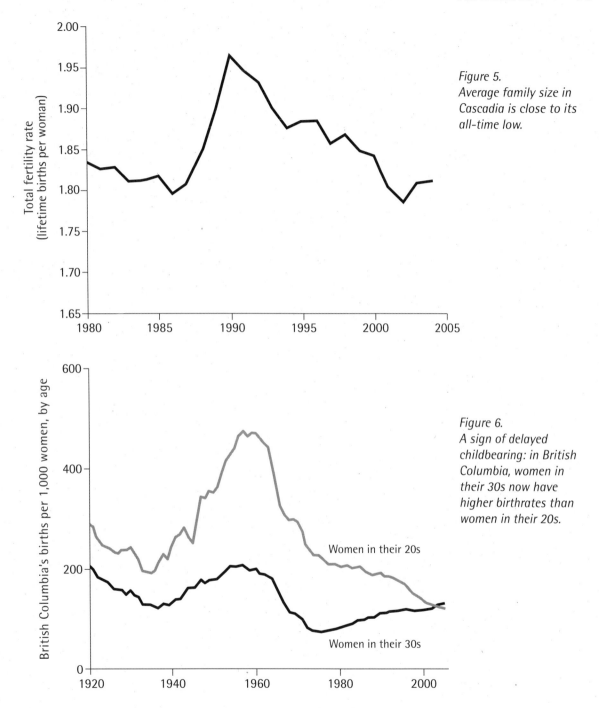

Figure 5.
Average family size in
Cascadia is close to its
all-time low.

Figure 6.
A sign of delayed
childbearing: in British
Columbia, women in
their 30s now have
higher birthrates than
women in their 20s.

for example, has roughly doubled in the last half century, to more than 26 percent in Oregon and Washington and 22 percent in Idaho.

As baby boomers become empty nesters (the oldest turn 60 in 2006), they promise to further expand the childless share of households. The over-65 cohort has grown slowly, from 10 percent to 12 percent of regional population since 1971, but it will rise to 20 percent by 2030 if government projections prove accurate. The region's under-15 cohort, meanwhile, has shrunk from 28 percent in 1971 to 19 percent in 2004. These trends in household composition bode well for the kinds of healthful, compact communities described in Chapter 6, "Special Section: Sprawl and Health."

Two recent trends in contraceptive access have helped women choose smaller, later families

Two recent trends in contraceptive access have helped women choose smaller, later families. First, insurance coverage for prescription contraceptives has improved markedly over the past decade. Thanks to new state laws and to lawsuits won by the Planned Parenthood Federation of Western Washington, the share of US employer-paid health plans with prescription drug benefits that pay for all prescription contraceptives soared from 28 percent in 1993 to 86 percent in 2002. In California and Washington, all such plans must do so, by state rule. Enacting similar rules in other Cascadian states would prevent thousands of unplanned pregnancies each year. Insurance coverage for prescription contraceptives increases the share of couples who use the most effective forms of contraception, such as the pill.

Second, emergency contraceptive pills are available from pharmacies without a doctor's prescription in Alaska, California, British Columbia, and Washington. (In one year, the advent of pharmacy access in British Columbia doubled the number of women using emergency contraception as a backup, usually for a torn or slipped condom.)

Oregon's senate, but not the state house, voted to add Oregon to this list in 2005. To expand these gains, the US Food and Drug Administration (FDA) can, like its Canadian and British counterparts, approve emergency contraceptives as nonprescription medication. The FDA's own scientists and outside peer reviewers have recommended doing so. As of early 2006, unfortunately, the agency had indefinitely postponed a decision on the proposal.

Although contraceptive access has improved, nearly 40 percent of births in the Northwest states still result from mistimed and unwanted pregnancies. Preventing such pregnancies has a range of powerful, compounding benefits. Children conceived intentionally are healthier: they receive better prenatal care and are less likely to have dangerously low weights at birth or to die in infancy. They also display superior verbal development in their early years and are less apt to endure abuse and neglect. Consequently, fewer wanted children end up in the child welfare system, including juvenile courts and foster care. By easing population pressures and reducing average family size, reductions in unintended pregnancy also gently reinforce the development of complete, compact communities, while reducing the aggregate consumption of natural resources. A goal of ensuring that every child is born wanted would mark a substantial contribution to the region's well-being. The slow-moving shift toward smaller, later families is a mark of progress toward this goal.

3. ENERGY

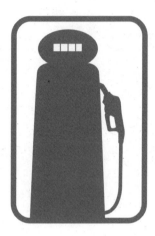

Energy consumption casts a long shadow over Cascadia. Hydropower dams have profoundly altered the region's rivers, while northwesterners' enormous appetite for fossil fuels contributes to global climate change and drains money from local economies to pay for energy imports. Cascadia's energy system also exposes the region to profound security vulnerabilities, some of which were highlighted in *Cascadia Scorecard 2005*. But 2005 contained a glimmer of promise for energy conservation: despite an uptick in the region's economy, per-person energy consumption remained flat and even declined slightly in the Northwest states (see Figure 7).

The Cascadia Scorecard tracks consumption of highway fuels and commercial and residential electricity as proxies for the larger trend of total energy use. Over time, these proxies have closely mirrored trends in overall energy use; and data for these trends are updated sooner and more reliably than some other components of the region's energy portfolio.

Despite high and rising gasoline prices through much of 2005, total gasoline use increased slightly from the previous year. Still, the aggregate use of gasoline in Cascadia has barely budged since 1999, even as population grew by 7 percent. As a result, per-person gasoline consumption fell by roughly 1 percent per year from 1999 to 2005 (see Figure 8). From a longer perspective, per capita gasoline consumption reached a plateau in the early 1980s, where it has remained fairly constant for more than two decades. The reduction in gasoline use that started in 1999 has been modest, but it may herald a new trend of declining personal consumption.

While the signs of improving fuel efficiency are welcome, the rising oil prices that sparked the reductions served as a stark warning. Even though

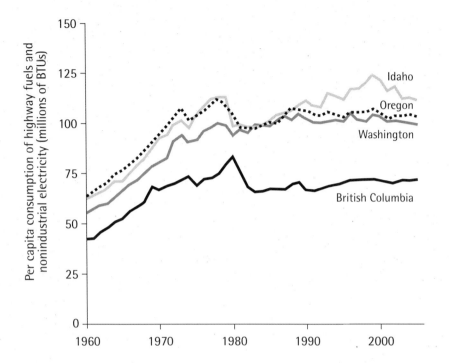

Figure 7.
Although energy use
in Cascadia declined
slightly in 2005,
it's been stuck at
a high plateau
since the 1980s.

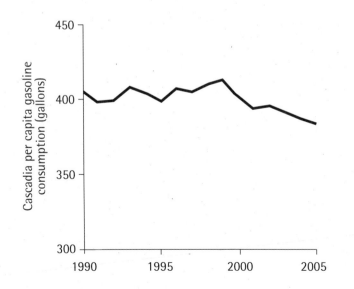

Figure 8.
Personal gasoline
consumption in
Cascadia has fallen
since 1999, most
likely because of
price increases.

The region has a host of options, both existing and on the near horizon, to reduce its oil dependence

much of the gasoline and diesel that power northwesterners' vehicles originated in nearby Alaska and Alberta, the price Cascadians pay for oil is determined in a global marketplace. Faraway events, including war in the Middle East, rising demand from the developing world, and supply disruptions caused by hurricanes in the Gulf of Mexico, pushed gasoline prices to record highs. The events of 2005 reminded northwesterners that their reliance on imported petroleum has made the region's economy vulnerable to forces over which residents have no control.

And despite recent reductions, Cascadians are still prodigious consumers of highway fuels: a typical northwesterner consumed more than a gallon of gasoline per day in 2005. But consumption patterns vary widely within the region. Residents of British Columbia continued to consume far less gasoline per person—roughly 5.3 gallons per week—than their neighbors to the south (see Figure 9). Typical residents of Oregon and Washington consumed roughly 8 gallons per week, while Idahoans averaged 8.7. But even Idaho's relatively high levels of consumption were lower than the US national average of 9 gallons per week per person. British Columbia's lower consumption is largely a result of the province's more compact communities and smaller road network—features that also benefit residents' health (see Chapter 6, "Special Section: Sprawl and Health"). Per resident, Washington has a quarter more miles of streets and highways than does British Columbia; Oregon has two-thirds more; and Idaho has three times more, which helps explain Idaho's comparatively high levels of highway-fuel consumption.

Even as per capita gasoline use declined, highway consumption of diesel fuel, which is used primarily for heavy truck transport, rose. In 2005 residents of the Northwest states consumed 2.4 gallons of diesel per week, while British Columbians used roughly 50 percent less. As with gasoline, Idaho is the Northwest's biggest per capita consumer of diesel, using one-third more than the US average.

The region has a host of options, both existing and on the near horizon, to reduce its oil dependence. Hybrid gasoline-electric vehicles,

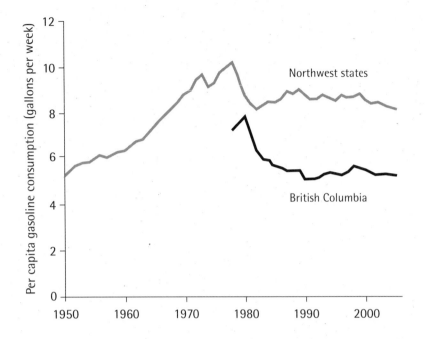

Figure 9.
Residents of
the Northwest
states use about
60 percent more
gasoline than
British Columbians.

as well as more efficient conventionally powered cars, have already begun to contribute to gasoline conservation. So-called plug-in hybrids, which use both gasoline (or gasoline-ethanol blends) and electricity from household outlets, can reduce petroleum consumption still further. And many researchers posit a future of lightweight but safe vehicles that could double fuel economy compared with today's models. Likewise, the advent of a cellulosic ethanol industry, using crop residues and other agricultural waste to generate transportation fuel, could foster energy independence while further reducing the region's greenhouse-gas emissions.

But if recent history is any guide, improved technology may not, by itself, curb Cascadia's appetite for highway fuels. Although vehicles are better engineered than they were in 1990, they are no more fuel efficient; as engine technology advanced, Cascadia's car buyers opted for larger and more powerful vehicles rather than more economical ones. Over the long run, policy changes may prove more effective than new technologies at jump-starting fuel conservation. For example, a system of vehicle "feebates"—levying sales charges on gas guzzlers to fund rebates on efficient models—would immediately boost the fuel economy of new vehicles. Likewise, fostering transit- and pedestrian-friendly neighborhoods can help residents cut their driving by half or more, without any changes in the vehicle fleet.

Residential and commercial electricity use in Cascadia remained roughly flat in 2005. As with highway fuels, British Columbia has the region's lowest demand for electricity in homes and businesses, using about one-fifth less per person than the Northwest states. Washington, Oregon, and Idaho all exceed the national average for electricity use, likely because a history of cheap electricity fostered installation of power-hungry appliances such as space heaters and electric water heaters.

Opportunities to reduce the impacts of Cascadia's electricity consumption abound. Energy-saving products, from compact fluorescent light bulbs to superefficient home appliances, are already proving their worth in homes and businesses. Renewable electricity generation—especially from wind and to a lesser extent from the sun—is well established in the region and has the potential to blossom given the right policy environment. Northwest researchers are also leading the way in developing "smart grid" systems, which use information technology to optimize the efficiency of electricity distribution and consumption while reducing the risk of power failures. Perhaps most powerfully, some utility oversight boards now allow electricity suppliers to make more money when they sell less power, a step that powerfully aligns utilities' incentives (higher profits) with consumers' (lower bills).

With wise decisions about policy and steady advancements in technology, Cascadia can extend its energy successes in 2005 to the years beyond. A healthier energy system would allow Cascadians to maintain their standards of living while reducing their consumption, and there is mounting evidence that this can be done.

A system of vehicle "feebates" would immediately boost the fuel economy of new vehicles

4. WILDLIFE

Cascadia Scorecard 2006 introduces a new measure of the health of our natural heritage: population trends for five emblematic wildlife species found in parts of the region. These include gray wolves in Idaho and western Montana; the Selkirk herd of mountain caribou; Oregon's greater sage-grouse; the southern resident orcas of Puget Sound and the Strait of Georgia; and chinook salmon that return to the lower Columbia River.

If Cascadia's forests, deserts, streams, and coasts are healthy and thriving, the region's salmon, orcas, gray wolves, caribou, and sage-grouse will thrive too. If not, they will dwindle and disappear. Like canaries in a coal mine, these five species point to early warnings of danger for humans too. They are also magnificent and fascinating exemplars of the natural inheritance that all Cascadians hold in trust.

In previous editions of the Cascadia Scorecard, trends in forest clear-cutting—as detected by satellite imagery—served as the rough-and-ready gauge for the status and trends in nature. Satellite data on deforestation appeared to be a reliable and timely indicator of the ongoing interaction between Cascadia's human inhabitants and the region's defining ecosystem. But the main satellite is malfunctioning badly, making a reliable and comprehensive update impossible.

Animals that once inhabited much of North America have been severely reduced in number (see Figure 10) as they have been confined to islands of protected habitat and to the northern reaches of their native ranges. Grizzly bears, for example, one of the Northwest's most awe-inspiring creatures, cling to a small portion of their former home (see map, page 39).

In 2006 the wildlife indicator reveals that there is reason for optimism about the state of the Northwest's natural systems. Several species that make up the wildlife indicator are showing promising resilience. But new threats also loom, including climate change and population pressure. Wildlife will not flourish in the coming decades without meaningful dedication to both conservation and restoration.

Figure 10. Although wildlife populations vary considerably, the five species measured by the Scorecard are well below their historic abundance.

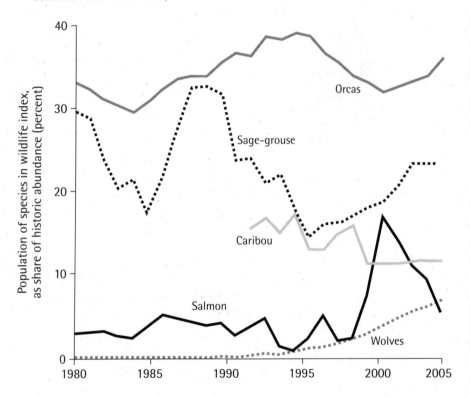

SALMON

Other than humans, no creature penetrates the Pacific Northwest as thoroughly as salmon. The wildlife indicator tracks spring and summer chinook salmon returning as adults to the Bonneville Dam, the lowest dam on the Columbia River and gateway to the vast hydrological system that binds British Columbia, Washington, Oregon, and Idaho.

Because of salmon's ubiquity, they may be the single best indicator of the Northwest's biological health. Changes in their populations can reflect any number of human influences, including dams, irrigation, clearcutting, suburban development, industrial waste, and global climate change, just to name a few. And just as salmon numbers are affected by a variety of factors, so their population fluctuations in turn have a profound effect on the health of dozens of species of birds, marine mammals such as orcas and sea lions, and even people.

Salmon once ranged throughout the Northwest, but at the region's southern end, where pressure from people is most intense, the percentage of imperiled wild stocks climbs (see map, page 40).

The chinook salmon report card is typical of the fate of salmon in the southern reaches of Cascadia. In recent years, chinook had returned to the Columbia in record numbers. But 2005 marked a return to the depressed levels typical of the 1980s and 1990s: roughly 150,000 fish, or less than 6 percent of their historic abundance. Returns in any single year are not an accurate measurement of long-term trends in salmon, because annual population counts vary widely (by an average 38 percent per year at Bonneville Dam). Though favorable ocean conditions may be responsible for the salmon boom years of the early twenty-first century, recent gains likely represent an improvement in conditions for salmon.

The real story of Columbia salmon, however, is much worse than the raw numbers suggest: most salmon on the Columbia are hatchery-raised fish, anemic cousins of the stronger wild fish, which are better signals of ecosystem health. Wild chinook may persist at less than 3 percent of their historic numbers.

Restoring salmon requires a variety of steps. Foremost among them are removing some dams, such as those on the lower Snake River; reducing pollution in the Columbia and other Northwest rivers; and developing more accurate pictures of salmon health through more-robust biological studies of rivers and streams. Reducing reliance on hydropower, by shifting to alternative energy sources and emphasizing conservation, also frees up more water for salmon to migrate past dams (see Chapter 3, "Energy").

ORCAS

If any other species is as emblematic of the Northwest as salmon, it is the orca, the distinctive black-and-white killer whale that plies the region's inland marine waters. Though they migrate seasonally, the best-known orcas—the southern residents—principally inhabit Puget Sound and the Strait of Georgia.

Orcas are an important part of the Northwest's cultural and ecological heritage. Considered totemic by native peoples but pests by fishermen, orcas were victims of aquarium collectors and even shooting until they began to gain protections in the 1970s. While they are no longer victims of outright hostility, orcas still face many human-made threats such as water contamination, decreased salmon stocks, and stress from marine traffic.

Strict protection measures helped restore the southern resident orca population from 70 individuals in 1976 to about 90 in 2006. Researchers have confirmed 7 new orcas since October 2004—one of the biggest population increases since the whales have been closely monitored.

In spite of the baby boom, the southern resident population is only about one-third of historic levels. Living much of the year near population centers—Seattle, Tacoma, Victoria, and Vancouver—these iconic creatures absorb the impact of the Northwest's cities and industries. They are exposed to such high levels of toxic contamination, including PCBs and PBDEs, that scientists consider them among the most contaminated marine mammals on earth (Chapter 5, "Pollution," discusses PCBs and PBDEs). Making matters worse, orcas' dietary mainstay, salmon, are too scarce.

In November 2005, the US National Marine Fisheries Service placed the orcas under the protective umbrella of the Endangered Species Act.

The resulting protections should help maintain this population by galvanizing local jurisdictions and providing federal money for restoration. Northwesterners can aid the orcas by restoring salmon runs and cleaning up toxics, actions that benefit people as well as hundreds of other species that inhabit the Northwest.

WOLVES

Once ranging across nearly every landscape in North America, wolves were hunted, trapped, and poisoned so extensively that they were rendered extinct in the western United States. But in the 1990s, US Fish and Wildlife officials reintroduced small populations into the northern Rocky Mountains (see map, page 41).

South of Canada, wolves primarily inhabit two states in Cascadia—Montana and Idaho—and they are expanding their range. Because wolves are cornerstone species for entire ecosystems—essential for maintaining ecological balance—their return to the Northwest signifies not only a return to wildness but a return to healthier natural places.

Their numbers remain small, but wolves have successfully reestablished themselves in the Northwest states. In just ten years since reintroduction, the wolf population has boomed and their range has expanded dramatically. An estimated 1,020 wolves inhabited Wyoming, Montana, and Idaho in 2005, exceeding the most optimistic expectations of a decade ago. (Idaho and Montana, whose wolf populations are part of the Scorecard wildlife indicator, were home to some 768 wolves as of 2005; see Figure 11.) Though annual growth rates vary, the overall trend is strongly upward, and pioneer wolves are moving into remote parts of Oregon and Washington.

As they multiply, wolves are helping to restore native ecology. In Yellowstone National Park their effects on their surroundings are extensively documented. Elk, which browse on new growth, no longer linger by streams because wolves can more easily catch them there. As a result, streamside trees are growing back. In turn, the increasingly tree-shaded

Wolves' return to the Northwest signifies not only a return to wildness but a return to healthier natural places

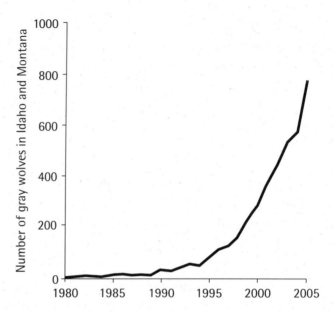

Figure 11.
Wolf reintroduction
in the northern
US Rockies has
been remarkably
successful.

streams support rebounding populations of native trout. Other plants flourish too, as do red foxes, beavers, and songbirds.

Unfortunately, proposals to remove wolves from the endangered species list would shift wolf management from federal to state authorities, making it easier to legally kill wolves before their populations can become firmly established in the Northwest.

To protect wolves, northwesterners can reexamine the mythology that mistakenly portrays wolves as hostile to people. We can instead welcome their return as agents of restoration. In addition, Oregon, Washington, and other largely wolfless places can consider reintroduction efforts of their own. Olympic National Park and surrounding wildlands are especially ripe: the park has stated that reintroducing wolves is a long-term management goal of the park, but that goal has languished since the 1990s.

CARIBOU

If wolves are the success story of the northern US Rockies, mountain caribou are the unfolding tragedy. Mountain caribou are the most endangered large mammal in the continental United States, and Cascadia is home to the last herd to venture south of the Canadian border. The Selkirk caribou inhabit the remote Selkirk Mountains of southeastern British Columbia, sometimes ranging south across the border into northeast Washington and northern Idaho.

Mountain caribou, a distinct "ecotype" of woodland caribou, require intact, mature mountain forests. Logging, road building, and development have constricted their food supply and habitat. Snowmobiles and other winter sports frighten the animals, keeping them out of their core habitat during lean winter months. Snowmobiles also leave packed routes in the snow, allowing predators to more easily penetrate backcountry caribou refuges. Finally, the herd has been harmed by an unintended chain reaction.

Over recent decades, the ecology of the Selkirk Mountains has become unbalanced. Clearcut logging destroyed prime forest habitat, robbing the caribou of their principal winter food sources. As the clearcuts also gave way to an abundance of tender regrowth, a favorite forage for white-tailed deer, the deer population exploded, but so did the population of formerly rare cougars, which prey on the deer. As a result, the caribou must contend with cougars.

Since 2000, the diminished Selkirk herd's population has hovered around 35 individuals, or roughly one-tenth of its historic number. The herd depends on a too-small established core reserve that protects them from snowmobiles and other disturbances. Officials credit recent population stability to liberal licensing of cougar hunts, which have depressed the local cat population and have given the caribou some breathing room. In the off-balance Selkirk ecosystem, a short-term reduction in the number of predators may be beneficial, at least to the caribou. But more important for the long-term survival of the caribou are intact wilderness-quality lands with old forests that support the animals' principal food sources.

Wildlife managers have augmented the herd several times by adding caribou from British Columbia's healthier herds. Without these infusions,

If wolves are the success story of the northern US Rockies, mountain caribou are the unfolding tragedy

the Selkirk caribou would probably have vanished. To date, the infusions have not returned the herd to viable size, so British Columbia is planning to transplant 60 new animals to the Selkirk herd. If predation stays low and human impacts are minimized, the Selkirk caribou may yet survive. Some officials in the province, however, have considered abandoning the Selkirk herd to concentrate restoration efforts on more stable caribou populations elsewhere in the province.

Even in British Columbia, where mountain caribou are more abundant, they are considered imperiled and their range has shrunk dramatically (see map, page 42), commensurate with expanded logging, development, and other habitat disruption in the Canadian Rockies.

The main chance for the Selkirk caribou to recover is through improved and expanded habitat, meaning strict protection and careful restoration of old-growth forests in the Selkirks. Older forests offer habitat and food for the caribou but constrain deer numbers, which in turn reduces predator populations. An easy first step would be expanding Washington's Salmo-Priest Wilderness, at the heart of the Selkirk herd's range, to include an adjacent 17,585-acre roadless area of national forest in Idaho.

The greater sage-grouse is a good indicator of an ecosystem once rich in native biological integrity

SAGE-GROUSE

Finally, the greater sage-grouse is a good indicator of an ecosystem once rich in native biological integrity that has been substantially diminished, both in extent and quality. As its name suggests, the sage-grouse depend on the sagebrush-dominated landscapes in the Northwest's dry interior country—in southern Idaho, eastern Washington, and eastern Oregon. Sightline's wildlife indicator monitors sage-grouse in Oregon, where their range is still fairly intact and where state biologists carefully track the bird's population.

As Lewis and Clark traveled through the Northwest in 1805 and 1806, they observed the birds in great numbers. But the succeeding two centuries have dramatically reduced sage-grouse numbers and have shrunk their range (see map, page 43). From building fences and transmission lines to mining and drilling, human activities affect the sage-grouse. Sagebrush eradication and expanding farms destroy habitat conspicuously, while livestock grazing and off-road vehicles accomplish the same end more subtly. Invasive species render sagebrush country more vulnerable to fire and simplify the native plant life, making the bird's food scarce.

Despite the extensive damage to their habitat, the sage-grouse populations in Oregon are oscillating within a stable range. Roughly 30,000 birds remain, which is probably less than 25 percent of historic levels. In Washington, only about 1,000 birds survive in two fragmented and vulnerable populations, a tiny percentage of their former abundance.

Returning sage-grouse populations to healthy levels will require coordinated ecological restoration as well as preservation of core habitat. Cascadia is home to several innovative success stories, including the Owyhee Initiative, a wildlands preservation project, in Idaho; the conversion of much of the Hanford Nuclear Reservation to conservation areas; and the banning of cattle from the Hart Mountain National Antelope Refuge in Oregon.

5. POLLUTION

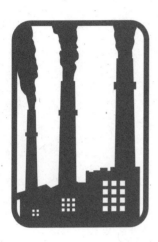

The Cascadia Scorecard's pollution indicator tracks levels of selected chemical contaminants in human bodies—the most intimate environment. Laboratory tests coordinated by Sightline Institute found chemical contaminants known as polychlorinated biphenyls, or PCBs, in each of 40 samples of breastmilk donated by Cascadian mothers. PCBs interfere with the immune system and hormone functioning and may retard intellectual development in children.

In some ways, the results of Sightline's tests were unremarkable: PCBs have been present in human tissues and body fluids for decades. But in another way, the findings were startling. With perhaps one exception, none of the women whose breastmilk was tested had worked in a job in which she might have been exposed to high levels of the contaminants. Food—typical grocery-store fare—was likely the main route of contamination for most study participants. And it should be cause for concern that the food supply still contains PCBs, as manufacture of the compounds was halted in the late 1970s, after their health effects on humans were documented. The PCBs that are present in our bodies and our foods represent a toxic legacy that is taking decades to fade.

PCBs are by no means the only contaminants of human manufacture that can be detected in northwesterners' bodies. Indeed, the body of every Cascadian resident, human and animal alike, contains a thin broth of products and by-products of modern industry, many of which did not exist a century ago. The most troublesome of these contaminants share three characteristics: they remain in the environment for years or decades after they are released; they accumulate in living things, including human bodies; and they are toxic, interfering with hormonal activity or other bodily functions, often at vanishingly small concentrations. Among these persistent bioaccumulative toxics are PCBs; flame retardants known as PBDEs; the long-banned pesticide DDT; and dioxins and furans.

Since the late 1970s, PCBs have been a dominant class of persistent bioaccumulative contaminants. Concentrations of PCBs have been significantly higher than chemically related contaminants, such as dioxins and furans. But recent trends suggest that concentrations of their chemical cousins, PBDEs, are rising rapidly and may be on the verge of overtaking PCBs in significance.

As reported in the 2005 edition of the Cascadia Scorecard, laboratory tests of breastmilk from the same 40 Cascadian mothers found PBDEs in each sample tested at levels 20 to 40 times higher than are commonly detected in northern Europe and Japan. The effects of PBDEs on laboratory animals are very similar to those of PCBs: laboratory animals exposed to the compounds early in life develop learning and behavioral aberrations that worsen with age.

On average, levels of PCBs still exceed those of PBDEs (see Table 2). Still, nearly one-third of the mothers in the study had higher levels of PBDEs than PCBs—a pattern that is emerging elsewhere in North America. And because PBDE contamination levels have been rising rapidly throughout Cascadia, the region may be fast approaching a point at which PBDEs outstrip PCBs as the persistent pollutant found at the greatest concentration in human bodies.

	Average PBDE level (parts per billion in breastmilk fat)	Average PCB level (parts per billion in breastmilk fat)
British Columbia	60	141
Montana	113	92
Oregon	121	187
Washington	88	300
Northwest (all)	96	190

Table 2. Levels of PCBs in the breastmilk of Northwest mothers still exceed those of PBDEs, but that's beginning to change.

Cascadians can reorient policies toward preventing contamination in the first place

Cascadia's high and rising PBDE levels suggest three courses of action. First, PBDE concentrations in human bodies should be closely tracked. North American production of the most troublesome forms of PBDEs ceased at the end of 2004, after the US Environmental Protection Agency reached an agreement with the main manufacturer to halt production. But this step will not guarantee that PBDE levels halt their meteoric ascent. As furniture foam and other consumer products age and degrade, they can release PBDEs into house dust, which may be a main source of contamination for people.

Second—particularly if levels of PBDEs continue to rise—Cascadia's governments should explore ways to remove the PBDEs that remain in people's homes and workplaces. The PBDE ban applies only to new products; it fails to address the risks from products that have already been manufactured and sold. Additional efforts will be required to rid people's homes of the compounds.

Third, and most importantly, Cascadians can reorient policies toward preventing contamination in the first place, rather than cleaning it up after the fact. In retrospect, it should have been obvious that PBDEs posed a hazard: their chemical structure is strikingly similar to that of PCBs and other well-recognized chemical threats. Had safety tests been performed before the compounds entered into commerce, we would not now have such cause for concern. Our treatment of untested chemicals has a pervasive flaw: we presume them innocent until proven guilty. As a result, we subject ourselves and our children to uncontrolled chemical experiments, discovering too late when the experiments have gone awry.

As with PCBs, there is no easy way to clean up the PBDEs that now lace our bodies; the chemical genie can't be put back in the bottle. But if we learn our lesson, we can avoid unleashing new chemical threats that could cloud our future.

6. SPECIAL SECTION: SPRAWL AND HEALTH

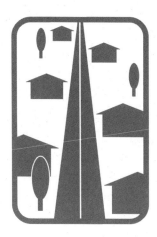

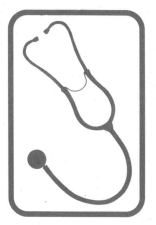

In 1943, British prime minister Winston Churchill stood before the assembled legislators of the House of Commons to recommend that their chambers, recently destroyed by an air raid, be rebuilt as they had once stood, essentially unchanged. To Churchill, the old hall's chief drawback—that it was too small to seat all its members—was actually a virtue. During critical votes, the overflowing aisles created an immediate, physical sense of urgency, which Churchill believed was precisely what such occasions demanded. Summing up his views, he remarked, "We shape our buildings; thereafter they shape us."

Much the same can be said of our cities and neighborhoods: we have shaped them, and now they are shaping us. Since the end of World War II, we have rebuilt our once pedestrian- and transit-friendly urban landscapes to accommodate the automobile. In relatively short order we laced our cities with superhighways and high-speed arterials; eliminated much of the network of streetcars that used to serve as mainstays of our public-transportation system; and encouraged the development of sparse, low-density suburbs at the urban fringe, a pattern of living that was once uncommon but for many has now become the norm.

More than 50 years into this new experiment in metropolitan form, our cities and suburbs are shaping us, but not always as we might hope. Low-density suburbs have their benefits, to be sure. But promoting exercise is not one of them: a lack of sidewalks, direct walking routes, and convenient nearby destinations turns walking from a form of transportation (taken regularly in small doses) into a form of recreation (taken irregularly, if at all). And by locking us into our automobiles for virtually every trip, sprawling land-use patterns not only promote sedentary lifestyles, but also expose residents to elevated risk of injury or death in car crashes.

The major cities of Cascadia serve as a de facto experiment concerning the effects of sprawl on health. The Canadian and US parts of the region exhibit very different patterns of urban and suburban land use, as well as substantial differences in human health. Those differences may be related: British Columbia's relatively strong record in controlling sprawl may have helped boost the province's health record.

BRITISH COLUMBIA: A LEADER IN HEALTH AND IN CURBING SPRAWL

Life expectancy in Cascadia rose slightly in 2003, the most recent year for which comprehensive, regionwide data are available. Given prevailing patterns of mortality, a newborn Cascadian could expect to live to just over 79 years, an increase of about two months over the previous year. Those increases have likely continued: in 2004, for example, Washington's life expectancy surged by 7 months. Still, British Columbia remains the region's life-expectancy leader, with lifespans in the province topping 81 years in 2005 (see Figure 12). If the province were an independent nation, its life expectancy would be the second highest in the world, trailing only Japan's.

Life expectancy is the best single measure of a region's health. It reflects everything that can hasten death, from infectious diseases to traffic accidents to cancer. It is statistically reliable and closely correlated with narrower measures of health, such as infant mortality and rates of preventable illness. And as a region's life expectancy lengthens, its residents typically spend more of their lives free from disability and satisfied with their health.

The gradual lengthening of lifespans—and improvement of overall health—has been a long-standing trend in Cascadia, as in the rest of the industrialized world. At the dawn of the twentieth century, a baby

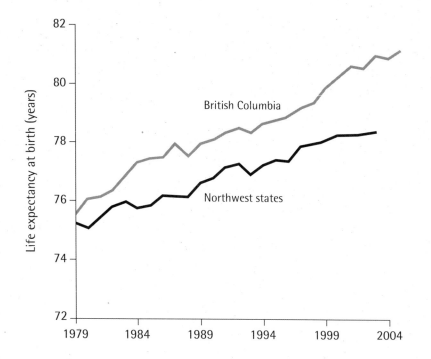

Figure 12.
The average lifespan
in British Columbia
now tops 81 years—
just behind the world
leader, Japan.

born in Cascadia could expect perhaps 50 years of life. Babies born at
the dawn of the twenty-first century could expect to live nearly three
decades longer—a greater increase in a single century than in all of prior
human history.

Cascadia's life expectancy has increased unevenly. At the end of the
1970s, British Columbia maintained only a three-month life expectancy
advantage over the Northwest states. Since that time, that lead has expanded to 2.5 years. At the recent pace of increase, it will take nearly
two full decades for the residents of Oregon, Idaho, and Washington
to match the longevity that BC residents already enjoy. By that point,
British Columbia will have extended its life expectancy lead over the
Northwest states to 4 years—roughly the same difference in lifespans
that currently separates the United States from Libya and Syria.

British Columbia's life-expectancy advantage appears to stem not
from a single cause but from many.

The province's health-care system is among the most significant contributors to British Columbia's health advantage. The provincial health-care system guarantees every resident access to basic medical care. In contrast, about 1 in 7 residents of the Northwest states go without any health insurance coverage for at least a year at a time. The province's health-care system saves money as well as lives; measured per resident, medical care costs nearly one-third less in British Columbia than in the Northwest states, despite the province's comprehensive coverage.

Medical care costs nearly one-third less per person in British Columbia than in the Northwest states

But while BC's universal health insurance certainly contributes to the province's superior health, it does not fully explain its longer lifespans. A 2002 report by the US National Academies' Institute of Medicine concluded that 18,000 US adults die each year because they lack health insurance. Those premature deaths shorten the average US lifespan by at most a few months. If that figure holds true for the two halves of Cascadia, then differences in access to health care explain a small fraction of the life-expectancy gap between British Columbia and the Northwest states. Clearly, British Columbia excels not only at providing health care once illness strikes, but also at preventing illnesses from occurring in the first place.

Demographic trends may also play a role in British Columbia's health advantage. The province has welcomed many new wealthy (and healthy) Asian immigrants over the past several decades, which may have boosted the province's longevity statistics. In contrast, the Northwest states' in-migrants tended to come from other parts of the United States, which ranks a disappointing 28th in life expectancy among all nations of the world—behind Cyprus, Costa Rica, and Chile. Compared with the rest of the United States, the Northwest states are relatively healthy, so in-migration likely did not boost the region's lifespans.

British Columbia also has lower infant mortality rates and fewer homicides than its southern neighbors. Still, none of these factors, singly or in combination, fully explain why BC residents live so much longer than their neighbors to the south.

As with health, British Columbia has a substantial advantage over the US Northwest in urban and suburban design—particularly in reining in low-density sprawl. Compared with Vancouver and Victoria, British Columbia, the major cities of Oregon, Washington, and Idaho are far more sparsely populated, with substantially fewer residents living in neighborhoods compact enough to allow some trips on public transit or on foot. Vancouver has been particularly successful at channeling new growth into compact, transit- and pedestrian-friendly communities. As with health, the province's lead in creating compact neighborhoods has widened in recent decades, with Vancouver leading the way (see Figure 13).

Vancouver's impressive record in promoting compact neighborhoods has been central to its excellent performance on a number of measures, including lower use of highway fuels (see Chapter 3, "Energy") and the preservation of agricultural land around cities. An emerging body of research also suggests that curbing sprawl may be lengthening British Columbians' lives.

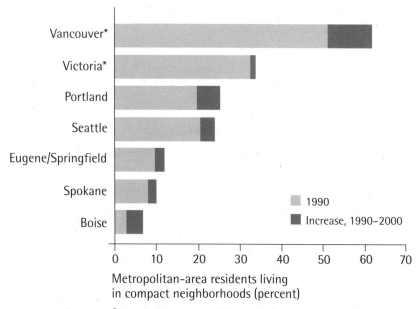

Figure 13. Vancouver, British Columbia, is far and away Cascadia's leader in creating compact communities.

Metropolitan-area residents living in compact neighborhoods (percent)

Data for Vancouver and Victoria are for 1991–2001.

Excessive sprawl can boost chronic illness by about the same amount as aging the entire city's population by four years

Put simply, this new research shows that sprawl can be hazardous to health. Comparisons of US metropolitan areas find that once income, education, and other relevant factors are taken into account, people living in sprawling areas tend to suffer substantially more chronic ailments—including diabetes, asthma, and hypertension—than people in more compact, transit- and pedestrian-friendly locales. Comparing cities with exceptional records in controlling sprawl with those that sprawl significantly more than average, the more-compact metropolises have about one fewer chronic illness for every ten residents. Said differently, excessive sprawl can boost chronic illness in a metropolis by about the same amount as aging the entire city's population by four years. Residents of the most sprawling counties are also more likely to be obese and physically inactive—and to suffer from high blood pressure—than are residents of the least sprawling counties.

Though available evidence suggests that sprawl worsens health, the precise mechanisms by which land-use patterns produce these effects are less certain. Most of the evidence suggests that the prime suspect in this health mystery is the automobile.

Day in and day out, residents of low-density sprawl log more miles in their cars than do people who live in more compact neighborhoods. Homes in sprawling suburbs tend to be surrounded by large yards, which create the "elbow room" that some residents cherish, but which also increase the distance between destinations. Zoning patterns in sprawling neighborhoods tend to keep residential and commercial areas strictly segregated, which makes walking inconvenient for most errands. This problem is compounded by the seas of parking surrounding many stores and workplaces, which further discourage walking. Branching suburban street design moves cars quickly onto expressways but also eliminates the direct routes from place to place that a traditional gridlike street layout provides.

These characteristics of sprawl—low-density housing, segregation of stores and homes, and lack of direct walking connections between destinations—substantially increase the distance that residents must

GRIZZLY BEAR: CURRENT AND HISTORIC RANGE

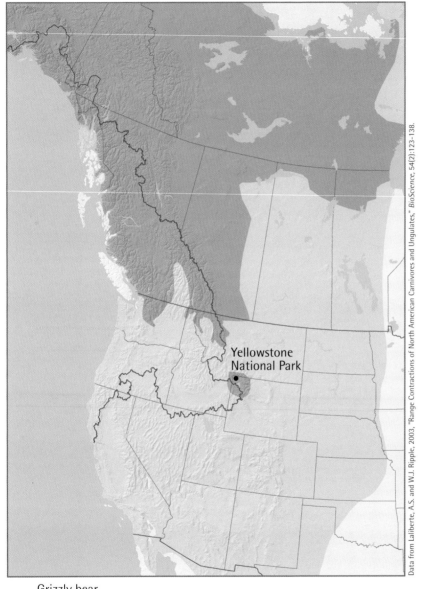

Data from Laliberte, A.S. and W.J. Ripple, 2003, "Range Contractions of North American Carnivores and Ungulates," *BioScience*, 54(2):123-138.

Yellowstone
National Park

Grizzlies once roamed throughout western North America, but their range has diminished substantially. All wildlife maps, except the salmon map, by CommEn Space.

Grizzly bear
 Range lost
Current range
— Cascadia boundary

SALMON: CURRENT ABUNDANCE IN CASCADIA

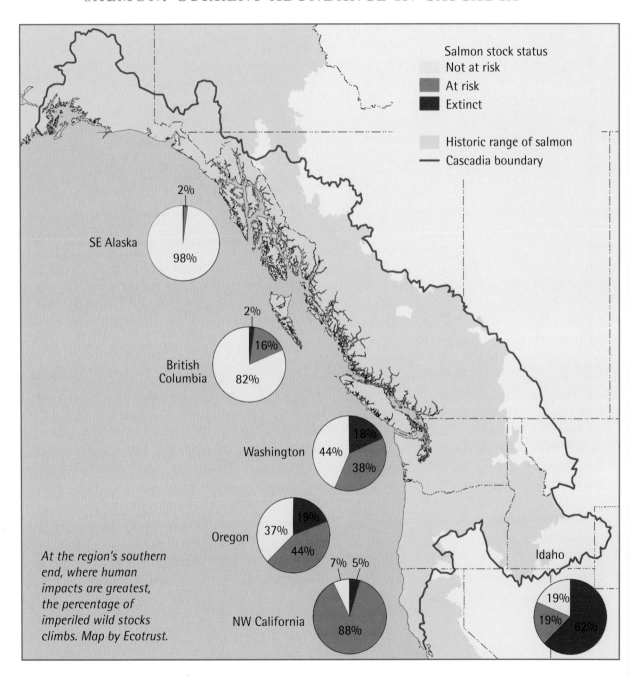

Salmon stock status
Not at risk
At risk
Extinct

Historic range of salmon
— Cascadia boundary

SE Alaska 2% 98%

British Columbia 2% 16% 82%

Washington 44% 18% 38%

Oregon 37% 19% 44%

NW California 7% 5% 88%

Idaho 19% 19% 62%

At the region's southern end, where human impacts are greatest, the percentage of imperiled wild stocks climbs. Map by Ecotrust.

GRAY WOLF: CURRENT AND HISTORIC RANGE

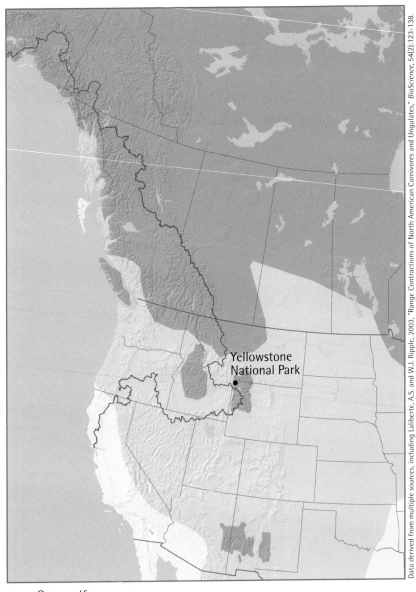

Data derived from multiple sources, including Laliberte, A.S. and W.J. Ripple, 2003, "Range Contractions of North American Carnivores and Ungulates," *BioScience*, 54(2):123–138.

Yellowstone
National Park

Despite recent population increases in Idaho, Montana, and Wyoming, gray wolves occupy only a small fraction of their historic habitat.

Gray wolf
Range lost
Current range
Cascadia boundary

TRAFFIC FATALITIES IN CASCADIA

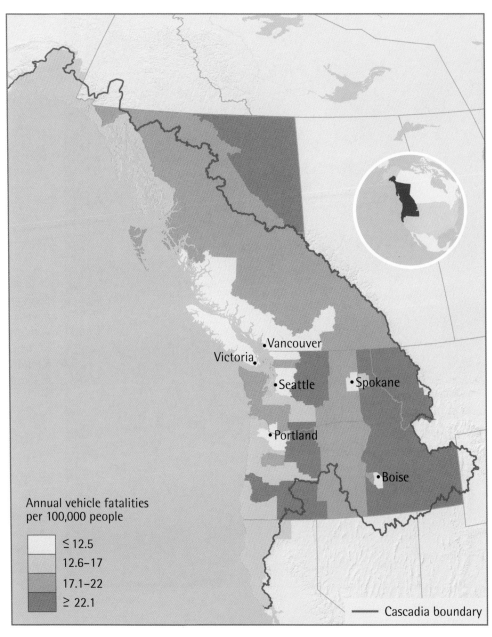

Annual vehicle fatalities
per 100,000 people

- ≤ 12.5
- 12.6–17
- 17.1–22
- ≥ 22.1

—— Cascadia boundary

Cascadia's urban areas, along with southwestern British Columbia,
excel at limiting the risk of car travel. Map by CommEn Space.

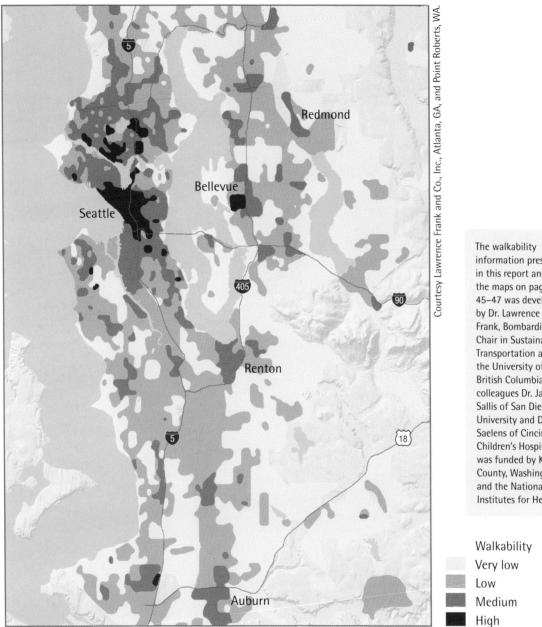

Courtesy Lawrence Frank and Co., Inc., Atlanta, GA, and Point Roberts, WA.

The walkability information presented in this report and in the maps on pages 45–47 was developed by Dr. Lawrence Frank, Bombardier Chair in Sustainable Transportation at the University of British Columbia, and colleagues Dr. James Sallis of San Diego State University and Dr. Brian Saelens of Cincinnati Children's Hospital, and was funded by King County, Washington, and the National Institutes for Health.

Walkability

Very low

Low

Medium

High

In King County, Washington, compact city and town centers promote walking, while sprawling suburbs discourage it. All transportation maps, except the traffic fatalities map, by Livni Consulting.

WHERE YOU CAN GO: A ONE-MILE WALK IN SEATTLE'S PHINNEY RIDGE NEIGHBORHOOD

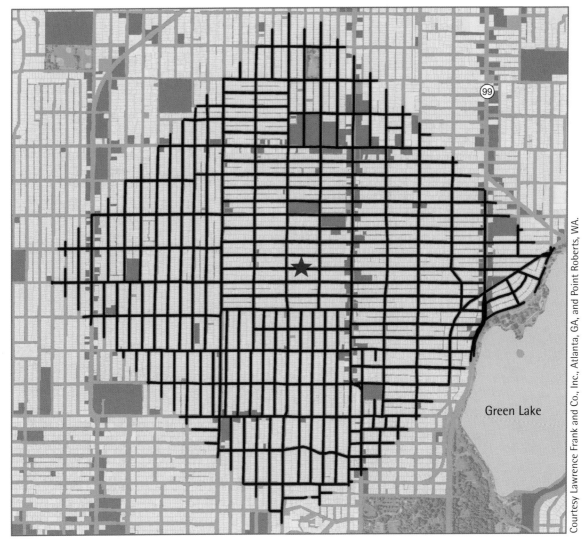

Green Lake

99

Courtesy Lawrence Frank and Co., Inc., Atlanta, GA, and Point Roberts, WA.

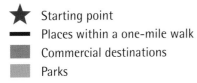

★ Starting point
— Places within a one-mile walk
■ Commercial destinations
■ Parks

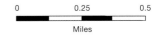

| 0 | 0.25 | 0.5 |

Miles

A gridlike street network with a mix of residences and businesses puts stores and services within a short walk of many homes; the blue lines illustrate destinations within a one-mile walking distance of the red star.

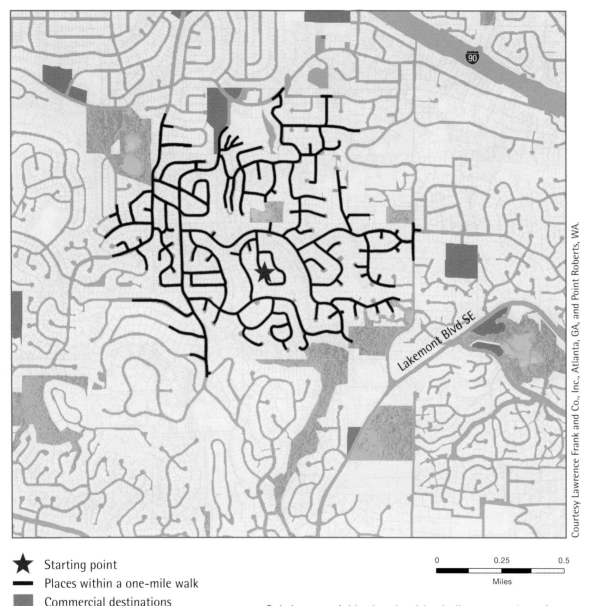

★ Starting point
▬ Places within a one-mile walk
■ Commercial destinations
▦ Parks

0   0.25   0.5
Miles

*Cul-de-sac neighborhoods with winding streets have few
commercial destinations within walking distance; the blue
lines illustrate destinations within a one-mile walking
distance of the red star.*

MORE MAPS, GRAPHICS, AND DATA AT SIGHTLINE.ORG

You can access animated versions of maps on our website at www.sightline.org. You'll also find print, Web, and PowerPoint versions of Scorecard maps and charts for your use; supplementary state, provincial, and local Scorecard data; and complete sources and citations.

travel to get to common destinations. In many sprawling neighborhoods, it is virtually impossible for residents to get around without a car; those without access to an automobile are stranded. In subtle yet cumulatively significant ways, extra driving adds to the burden of death, injury, and disease. Car accidents, obesity and physical inactivity, exposure to air pollution, and reduced opportunities for neighborly interactions can all result. And all these things take their toll on our health.

CAR CRASHES

The news is all too common, so the stories are often consigned to the inner pages of the local sections of Cascadia's newspapers. And the headlines—as shown by this small sampling from early 2006—give the merest hint of the tragedy that engulfs the victims and their families: "Two killed in vehicle accident," "Head-on crash east of Salem kills 3," "Veneta man dies in solo Hwy. 38 crash," "Driver sentenced 30 years for deaths of father and son," "Crash victim called 'great family man.'"

Car crashes pose a huge—and underappreciated—risk to Cascadians' health: a tragedy of epic scale, but one that fades from our attention because it unfolds only gradually, as if in slow motion. On average, collisions claim 5 lives each day across the region: 1 each, perhaps, in Oregon, British Columbia, and Idaho, and 2 in Washington. But over time this death toll mounts to staggering proportions. In all, some 50,000 Cascadians have perished in car crashes since 1980.

Measured by the mile or kilometer, traveling by automobile can seem fairly safe: Cascadia suffers just 1 traffic fatality for every 65 million miles (104 million km) driven. But Cascadians rack up a staggering number of miles in their cars and trucks—roughly 130 billion miles (210 billion km) each year. Mile after mile, the risk adds up, leading to an annual body count that approaches 2,000 lives lost.

Teens and young adults are particularly prone to accidents; traffic fatalities spike between the ages of 15 and 24. As a result, car crashes have become the leading cause of death under age 45 in Cascadia and trail only heart disease and cancer in shortening the lives of Cascadians under the age of 65. And because crashes often involve the young, they disproportionately shorten lifespans: Idaho's average life expectancy would lengthen by more than six months if car crashes could be completely eliminated.

Fatalities are only one part of the story of car crashes; vehicle injuries, from the minor to the disfiguring, are far more common. In the United States, the National Safety Council estimates that for each vehicle fatality, 52 people are injured in car crashes, some of them severely. Based on this rule of thumb, some 100,000 Cascadians sustain injuries in car crashes each year, with more than 2 million collision injuries sustained regionwide since 1980. Washington's transportation department places the injury rate even higher than the safety council's estimates, with collisions injuring some 47,000 state residents in 2002 (enough to fill the Safeco Field stadium, where the Seattle Mariners play), including 2,500 who suffered disabling injuries.

Injuries and loss of life are the most appropriate metrics by which to gauge the harm of car crashes, but economic measures provide added perspective. According to National Safety Council figures, each vehicle fatality corresponds to $5.2 million in economic costs, a figure that includes medical outlays, lost wages, forgone productivity, property damage, and administrative expenses. Using this figure, car crashes may drain the economies of Washington, Oregon, and Idaho of $8 billion per year—an annual tax of more than $700 per resident, or $1 for every $50 produced by the region's economy.

This estimate of the economic cost of car crashes is conservative. Washington's transportation department tallied comprehensive crash costs in the state at $930 per resident in 2002, or $5.5 billion total—which is more than three times the department's entire yearly budget. These figures suggest that car crashes may cost more than the roads on which they occur. Other estimates, based on how much people appear to be willing to pay to avoid injury or death, place the comprehensive cost of collisions higher still.

Perhaps surprisingly, it is in the densest urban places of Cascadia—the very places associated in the public mind with the worst congestion—that residents face the lowest risk of dying in a traffic accident. Residents of Vancouver's city center, for example, face a fatal crash risk one-third as high as the provincewide average. King County—the most urbanized county in Washington—and the home of Seattle, Bellevue, and other urban centers—has the lowest overall crash risk of any county in the state. Multnomah and Washington counties—the most urban parts of metropolitan Portland—lead the way in Oregon. And Ada County, home of Boise—the state's biggest city—has Idaho's lowest crash risk (see map, page 44).

Metropolitan areas across the United States show a similar pattern: the risk of dying in a transportation accident—combining deaths among pedestrians, transit riders, bicyclists, and occupants of cars and trucks—is consistently lower in compact metropolitan areas than in sprawling ones. Even pedestrians were safer in more densely populated places; walkers find safety in numbers, since drivers apparently adjust to sharing the road as the numbers of pedestrians and bicyclists rise.

City dwellers face low accident risk simply because they drive so little. Crash risk tends to be proportional to distance driven; all else being equal, the more one drives, the greater one's risk. Residents of sprawling neighborhoods drive longer distances, and spend more time overall in their cars, than do residents of more compact neighborhoods. Many residents of compact cities and suburbs can take transit for some trips, which yields an additional safety bonus: mile for mile, riding a bus is more than ten times safer than driving a car.

Compact neighborhoods protect drivers and pedestrians in other ways as well. Traffic on the narrow streets of cities and denser suburbs tends to move more slowly than on wide suburban arterials, lessening

Mile for mile, riding a bus is more than ten times safer than driving a car

the severity of collisions. A walker struck by a motor vehicle traveling at 40 miles per hour (64 kph) survives only 15 percent of the time. At 30 miles per hour (48 kph) the odds of survival rise to 45 percent. At 20 miles per hour they soar to 95 percent.

In Cascadia, differences in crash risk seem to account for some of the health gap between British Columbia and the Northwest states. On average, BC residents drive significantly less than their counterparts to the south—some 4,400 miles (7,100 km) less each year—largely because of the compact urban design of their major metropolitan areas. Overall, residents of Oregon, Idaho, and Washington face about a 45 percent greater risk of dying in a car crash than do British Columbians—which subtracts between one and two months from their lifespans. In economic terms, reducing crash fatalities in the Northwest states to the levels prevalent in British Columbia could give the region an economic lift of about $220 per resident in avoided medical expenses, productivity gains, and other costs of car crashes.

WALKING

The United States and Canada are in the midst of two concurrent and closely related epidemics: rising rates of obesity and falling levels of physical activity. Put simply, we are fatter than we used to be, and we get far less exercise than we should.

Obesity rates have more than doubled in the Northwest states just since 1990. More than 1 in 5 residents of Washington, Oregon, and Idaho now qualify as obese, while nearly an additional 4 in 10 are overweight. Obesity rates are rising particularly fast among children; in Washington State, one child in seven is obese. Meanwhile, nearly half of adults in the Northwest states fail to get even the recommended 30 minutes of moderate daily exercise. Obesity trends in British Columbia are moving in the same direction as in the Northwest states, though only about one-fourth as fast; still, about 1 in 9 residents of the province is obese.

Combined, the obesity and inactivity epidemics are having a profound effect on health. Obesity increases the risk of high blood pressure, heart disease, stroke, gallbladder disease, osteoarthritis, and cancers of the breast and colon, among other ailments. Physical inactivity has been linked with a similar range of maladies, as well as depression and anxiety. Both have contributed to the alarming rise in what was once called "adult onset" diabetes, which is now claiming an increasing number of children as victims.

The diseases brought on by obesity and inactivity shorten Cascadians' lives. The most recent estimates place the death toll from obesity in the United States at 112,000 per year, though previous estimates had been considerably higher. Based on obesity rates in the Northwest states, this suggests that obesity kills some 2,300 people per year in Washington, 1,500 in Oregon, and 540 in Idaho. Long-term studies suggest that obesity shortens lifespans and increases the risk of death from a large range of ailments. Some researchers even theorize that rising rates of obesity may eventually lead to a decline in US life expectancy, while others suggest that high obesity rates in the United States may explain Canada's substantial lead in life expectancy over its southern neighbor.

All told, the total costs of obesity and physical inactivity—combining medical outlays, workers' compensation expenditures, lower productivity, and other factors—probably top $11 billion per year in the Northwest states, or just under $1,000 per resident. Oregon, Washington, and Idaho spend a combined $2.3 billion annually for medical treatments related to obesity and an additional $1.4 billion to $3.4 billion for medical treatments related to physical inactivity. (The comprehensive costs of physical inactivity in British Columbia are thought to be somewhat lower, at Can$211 million annually.) Even more significantly, a physically inactive workforce tends to be less productive, which may sap an additional $8 billion from the economies of the Northwest states ($4.8 billion in Washington, $2.5 billion in Oregon, and $815 million

Obesity kills some 2,300 people per year in Washington, 1,500 in Oregon, and 540 in Idaho

in Idaho), as well as Can$362 million in output from British Columbia. Even small reductions in obesity and physical inactivity could boost the Northwest economy by hundreds of millions of dollars per year.

Both obesity and physical inactivity have many causes. The proliferation of sedentary jobs, passive recreation, and cheaper calorie-rich foods has played a role. So has the gradual decline in walking as a form of transportation—to work, to stores, even to friends' houses. And sprawling neighborhood design has discouraged walking.

Studies have found that residents of "walkable" neighborhoods are less likely to be obese than are residents of more-sprawling locales

Studies in Atlanta, Seattle, and Vancouver conducted by University of British Columbia's Lawrence Frank and colleagues, and a similar study in San Diego, found that residents of "walkable" neighborhoods—where stores and homes are mingled and streets form grid patterns that create direct routes between destinations—are less likely to be obese than are residents of more-sprawling locales. In Atlanta, for example, people who live in the least walkable neighborhoods are about a third more likely to be obese than residents of neighborhoods that best supported foot traffic. Similarly, San Diego residents who live in neighborhoods with ample pedestrian amenities walk more for errands, get ten extra minutes of physical activity per day, and are 40 percent less likely to be overweight than residents of sprawling neighborhoods. Frank's study in King County, Washington compared residents of high-walkability and low-walkability communities and found that pedestrian-friendly neighborhood design is associated with up to a one-point reduction in the body mass index, a measure of weight versus height. For someone who is 5 feet 9 inches tall (175 cm), living in a low-walkability neighborhood translates into up to 7 pounds (3 kg) of extra body weight. The most walking-friendly neighborhoods in King County were in and around dense city and town centers—places with interconnected streets as well as stores and services located near housing (see maps, pages 45–47).

Not only do residents of sprawling neighborhoods walk less than residents of more pedestrian-friendly places, but they also spend more time in their cars. A major US transportation survey shows that people who live in low-density suburbs spend an average of 20 more minutes each day in a car than do residents of the most compact neighborhoods. Research shows that on average, each additional hour a day spent in a car raises the likelihood of being obese by 6 percent.

Most studies find that neighborhood design boosts walking by only a few extra minutes per day, on average. But even small increases in daily exercise add up. Burning just ten extra calories per day—the amount burned during a two- to three-minute walk—can prevent a pound of weight gain per year. Compounded across decades, such small variations in daily exercise can easily make the difference in maintaining a healthy weight.

AIR

On a back street of Seattle's Beacon Hill, two miles southeast of downtown, sits a small building bristling with high-tech air quality sensors—one of a handful of such air-monitoring stations maintained in both urban and suburban locations around Puget Sound. The station's equipment measures fine particulate matter (including the carcinogenic soot that is a by-product of diesel combustion), ground-level ozone, volatile organic compounds (VOCs), and other common pollutants that have been linked to health problems ranging from asthma to cancer.

By virtually any reckoning, Beacon Hill should be a hot spot for polluted air. It is surrounded by freeways, industry, and giant container ships at dock. But the Beacon Hill monitoring station typically registers good news, even compared with its suburban counterparts. It registers less ozone than any other monitoring station in the region, and its carbon monoxide levels are the lowest among the six stations that monitor the compound, with peak concentrations about 45 percent lower than at several monitoring stations far from the city center. Levels of volatile organics and airborne metals are a bit high, but for fine particulate matter Beacon Hill does moderately well: third best of 7 regional monitoring stations by one measure, seventh of 16 by another, best among 5 by yet another. Beacon Hill residents can certainly hope for better air quality, and the pollution that does exist likely exacerbates asthma and other ailments among the neighborhood's residents. But all in all—and especially compared with the levels of pollution that might be expected given the neighborhood's location—people who live on Beacon Hill have cause to breathe a sigh of relief.

Beacon Hill exemplifies a surprising fact about air quality in the Pacific Northwest's metropolitan areas: suburban air is not necessarily cleaner than the air in urban neighborhoods. Whether a neighborhood's air is clean or dirty depends on hard-to-predict factors, such as prevailing weather patterns and the precise location of major pollution sources. Rules of thumb—such as whether a neighborhood is near a highway or industrial zone, in a city center or a leafy suburb—go only so far. Indeed, among monitoring stations in the Northwest states, those in suburban areas tend to record slightly higher levels of soot, dust, and smog than those in urban places. One reason is that emissions from the cities tend to migrate outward to the suburbs—and can actually get worse en route. Smog, for example, is formed through the interaction of sunlight with certain kinds of emissions, which means that smog precursors that are released near a city center may turn into lung-irritating smog only after they have drifted out to the suburbs. This helps explain why the highest levels of smog in the greater Puget Sound area are found in North Bend and Enumclaw, towns and suburbs that are far from the urban core.

Overall, the Northwest's air is cleaner than it used to be. No longer do health experts compare breathing the air in downtown Portland to smoking a pack of cigarettes a day, as they did in the 1960s. Similarly, the number of unhealthy air days in Washington State—days when at least one federally regulated air pollutant exceeded health limits—declined from a high of 150 days in 1987 to just 7 days in 1999—a 20-fold decline in just 12 years. Stricter laws, shifts in industry, and fewer logs on the hearth have all cleared the air somewhat, but perhaps most important, today's cars are far cleaner than their predecessors. They emit virtually no lead and dramatically less other pollution as well.

But while cars are cleaner than they were two decades ago, they are also busier and more numerous. As a result, motor vehicles remain the single largest source of air pollution in Cascadia's urban areas. In a typical year of driving, a single car or truck emits about a quarter of its weight in the most troublesome air pollutants, including lung-harming smog precursors, plus twice its weight in emissions that contribute to global warming. These emissions add up quickly. In Washington State, for example, motor vehicles generate nearly three-fifths of all federally regulated air pollution in the state—pollutants that contribute to asthma, lung disease, and cancer. Environmental contaminants, including pollution from cars, take more than $600 million out of the pockets of Washington residents to pay medical expenses and other costs associated with asthma and cardiovascular disease.

Polluted air, not surprisingly, is commonplace along the busiest highways: in fact, crowded highways are like "tunnels of pollution." This means that the air in heavy traffic is the most polluted air that many people breathe all day. It can trigger abnormal heart rhythms, lung inflammation, and other ailments. A tragic irony follows from these facts: people who seek fresh air by living in distant suburbs may actually wind up breathing worse air because of the pollution inside their vehicles.

Suburban residents also generate more air pollution on average. A study of the travel habits of King County residents, by University of British Columbia's Lawrence Frank and colleagues, found that people who live in the most sprawling, low-density suburbs—locales with poorly connected street networks and little intermixing of stores and homes—drive substantially more than people in more pedestrian- and transit-friendly neighborhoods. And more driving means more pollution: compared with residents of compact neighborhoods, residents of sprawling suburbs generate about one-quarter more ozone-forming nitrogen oxides and slightly more volatile organic compounds in a typical day of driving.

In Washington State, motor vehicles generate nearly three-fifths of all federally regulated air pollution—pollutants that contribute to asthma, lung disease, and cancer

COMMUNITY

Friendship can be powerful medicine, as study after study shows. Strong and regular ties to confidantes and community safeguard health, helping many people—particularly men and the elderly—weather disease. Conversely, people who are socially isolated are more likely to get sick or die. So strong is the effect of social companionship on health that a lack of community ties can be as harmful to health as smoking, obesity, high cholesterol, or physical inactivity.

Friendship, trust, and community ties are not simply relationships among individuals; they are rooted in a phenomenon known to researchers as "social capital," a term used to describe the strength and character of the bonds among family, friends, neighbors, and even strangers. Levels of social capital have been in steady decline in the United States since the 1950s. Based on proxies such as membership in community organizations, church attendance, and voter participation, it appears that social capital has ebbed to its lowest level since useful records have been kept.

The gradual unraveling of social bonds in the United States may be shortening our lives. Residents of states with high levels of interpersonal trust (a sign of high social capital), for example, tend to report better health. Conversely, in states where people think others will take advantage of them (a signal of low social capital), residents tend to have higher mortality rates. Low social capital has also been linked with higher rates of violent crime, binge drinking, teen pregnancies, and depression and with lower rates of leisure-time physical activity. All of these factors point to high levels of social capital as a strong corollary—and perhaps a cause—of a healthy population. ·

Poorly planned development may be partly responsible for the decline in social capital in the United States. Compact neighborhoods can foster casual social interactions among neighbors, while low-density sprawl creates barriers to such neighborly ties.

Sprawl tends to replace public spaces such as parks with private spaces such as fenced-in backyards, which reduce opportunities for informal socializing. Low-density development can physically separate neighbor from neighbor, limiting the casual interactions that help create a sense of community. And residents of sprawling neighborhoods rarely walk for transportation, which reduces opportunities for face-to-face contact with neighbors. One study of three US cities found that, in areas with a relatively high share of drive-alone commuters, residents are less likely to have close social ties within their own communities. Studies have also found that for each ten additional minutes a person spends in a daily commute, the time spent involved in community activities falls by 10 percent.

Conversely, pedestrian-friendly community design seems to help foster neighborhood ties. A comparison of two demographically similar neighborhoods in Portland, Oregon, found that a safe and interesting walking environment was linked with higher levels of social capital. Another study in Galway, Ireland, came to similar conclusions: neighborhoods that foster walking have higher social capital. Mixed-use neighborhoods that support both residential and commercial development can also increase opportunities for spontaneous social interaction and incidental contact. However, compact neighborhood design can backfire: several studies have found that very high residential density may be linked with a reduced sense of community.

Compact neighborhoods with a mix of housing types—single-family homes, multifamily housing, and even elder housing—may have an additional benefit for health. Diversified housing can meet the housing needs of residents over many stages of life, whether as singles, families, or empty nesters. And this in turn can allow aging residents to remain in their communities, maintaining connections with friends and neighbors. Maintaining such social ties can be particularly effective at buoying the health of the elderly.

Diversified housing can meet the housing needs of residents over many stages of life

Evidence about the connections among neighborhood design, social capital, and health is not yet complete. Still, research suggests that compact communities may help insure us against the ill effects of social isolation.

CHOICES

Step by step, the extra walking helps the family in the compact neighborhood remain, well, compact

Two families each choose a new home in the same metropolis. One family elects a far-flung area at the rural fringe, where it can afford a large house with a large yard. This neighborhood has no sidewalks and few destinations within walking distance. Virtually every trip requires a car, so the family decides that each driver needs a separate vehicle. And since it is quite a drive to stores and jobs, each car (or truck) racks up more than 10,000 miles per year.

The other family chooses a smaller home, closer to a town or city center and with stores and services nearby. Family members still make most trips by car, but the trips tend to be shorter. They log fewer miles in their cars, and they are able to walk to some errands. They even ride the bus occasionally—which lets them get by without a car for every driver in the household.

The two families' lives are similar. They both spend about the same amount of time traveling from place to place, and they both take most of their trips in a car or truck. The differences are small: members of the family in the more pedestrian-friendly neighborhood spend an extra half hour walking each week. They drive one-third fewer miles.

But over time, these differences compound. Step by step, the extra walking helps the family in the compact neighborhood remain, well, compact. They keep off weight and exercise more, helping to prevent chronic ailments such as diabetes and heart disease. Fewer miles in cars—and perhaps more in buses—keep them safer from fatal or debilitating crashes. The air they breathe may even be cleaner than their suburban counterparts', especially if they spend less time in the "pollution tunnel" of busy highways. And they may interact with their neighbors more, which helps connect them to their community and fosters close friendships within their own neighborhood. This in turn may help buoy their health and lift their spirits in hard times.

Conversely, the family in the sprawling neighborhood is more prone to weight gain and inactivity (and the resulting disease) and car and truck crashes (and the resulting devastation). They spend more time in their cars, which may expose them to worse air quality on the highway, while diminishing their contacts with neighbors and involvement in their community.

The difference between the families on any of these measures would not be large. But small differences spread across millions of such families amount to colossal costs: sprawl cuts short Cascadians' lives.

CONCLUSION:
A HEALTHY PLACE

In the late summer of 1854, physician John Snow, confronted by a rampant cholera epidemic in a London neighborhood, hit upon a remedy that was as remarkable for its simplicity as for its effectiveness: he asked local officials to remove the handle of a public water pump located at the epicenter of the outbreak. In an era when contagion was still poorly understood, Snow was convinced that the water from that pump contained a cholera pathogen. Removing the pump handle, he reasoned, would be the easiest and fastest way to halt the disease's spread. The officials agreed to act on Snow's recommendations, and perhaps half an hour of labor sufficed to save dozens or even hundreds of lives.

This episode has become legendary in the fields of public health and epidemiology, for it embodies two critical insights: first, that preventing disease can be far easier than curing it; and second, that complex problems sometimes have simple—though not necessarily obvious—solutions.

Creating a healthier place—where people are more satisfied with their lives, less encumbered by illness, and surrounded by thriving nature—is undoubtedly more complicated than stopping a neighborhood cholera outbreak. It involves a gradual realignment of many policies and institutions, both public and private, as well as reformation of deeply ingrained habits and outlooks. But perhaps the most effective way to approach the task is to identify the simple, often unheralded steps that, like Snow's pump handle, employ modest means to achieve far-reaching ends.

The connection between urban design and health is perhaps the best such example from this year's Scorecard. Not only is sprawl among the Scorecard's worst-performing indicators, it is also a root cause of some of the Northwest's most troubling ills, making it a drag on other indicator scores. Sprawling, poorly planned development contributes to the Northwest's vast appetite for gasoline and diesel fuel. It strains the economy to pay for fuel imports and to build and maintain cars and roads. It entails the gradual paving of both farmland and natural lowland habitats, which frays both terrestrial and aquatic ecosystems. And as the previous chapter shows, sprawl increases driving-related health risks from car crashes, obesity, and vehicle emissions. Finding simple policy changes that promote and nourish complete, compact communities—the opposite of poorly planned sprawl—could yield compounding benefits both for Cascadia's human inhabitants and for the natural systems that support them.

There is no one single solution to sprawl, but there are a number of modest steps that, taken together, could draw development away from the urban fringe and toward the established and growing city and town centers across the major metropolises of the Northwest. These steps require no new technologies or expensive investments, relying instead on modest alterations to the rules and systems that govern land use and transportation decisions throughout the region.

- **When building roads, budget for health.** As a transportation agency prepares to build a new road, it budgets assiduously for construction costs such as labor, land, and materials. But the increased car crashes and other health costs that result from road building do not appear in the agency's ledgers. These costs are passed along to taxpayers and society at large, whether as higher medical bills, higher taxes to pay for government services, or— for those directly harmed—lower quality of life. Since these costs are not accounted for at the time that transportation projects are planned, they are invisible to the people most responsible for transportation decisions.

If transportation planners were required to incorporate—or simply to investigate—comprehensive health costs when making budgeting decisions, they might well discover that some projects simply do not merit the expense. Road projects, particularly those at the edges of metropolitan areas, might seem cost-effective on their face, but factoring in the extra traffic accidents and obesity-inducing sprawl that follows in the wake of many new roads can make them seem like expensive boondoggles. Also, a comprehensive assessment of the health benefits of pedestrian infrastructure, traffic safety, or transit investments might well find that these are surprisingly cost-effective because of their attendant benefits on health. Simply revealing what is hidden—the true costs and benefits of transportation projects—can ensure that the region makes wiser and more health-promoting transportation decisions.

- **Zone for life.** After World War II—when vehicle ownership was becoming widespread—public-health officials raved about the health benefits of leafy suburbs. And rightly so. Soot and industrial fumes clouded the air in many cities and town centers, and even though traffic congestion was less prevalent then than it is now, automobile exhaust was more hazardous. Escaping to the greener spaces on the urban fringe seemed a healthy choice. Partly as a consequence, zoning rules and related policies encouraged—and in some cases even required—low-density suburbs, with homes surrounded by large yards and segregated from stores and workplaces.

  Today, however, the tables have turned. Places that are compact enough to foster walking and biking—the modern (and cleaner) city and town centers once shunned by enlightened planners—now tend to be healthier places to live than sprawling, low-density suburbs. But our policies have not changed to reflect this reality. Many locales still mandate low-density housing while restricting infill development and accessory dwelling units (sometimes called "granny flats") which can help more people live in the most pedestrian-friendly neighborhoods. Likewise, local land-use rules often require developers to provide overabundant parking, which makes commercial development more expensive while spreading destinations farther apart. And traffic codes—along with the engineering profession itself—still favor branching street networks that impede short trips to nearby destinations.

Changing zoning and transportation policies is, admittedly, slow work. But as Vancouver, British Columbia's smart-growth record shows, government policies that promote higher-density development can, over the long term, be surpassingly effective at channeling growth. Thousands of Cascadians are already working to change how their communities grow—to lift onerous parking requirements, allow infill development in already developed areas, encourage a mix of stores and services in residential zones, and create development boundaries that help keep growth from spiraling outward into farms and forests. Seattle's "center city" strategy is one example of a policy change that is helping to foster new residences within walking distance of downtown. As more voices speak out about the health benefits of curbing sprawl, this trend is likely to accelerate.

Seattle's "center city" strategy is one example of a policy change that is helping to foster new residences within walking distance of downtown

- **End subsidies that accelerate sprawl.** In ways that are both obvious and subtle, tax codes and government spending priorities tilt in favor of low-density development at the urban fringe and against redevelopment in already established neighborhoods.

  For example, developers rarely pay the full cost for the public infrastructure—roads, sewer and water lines, schools, police and fire stations, and the like—that services the most sprawling, low-density development. Even the "impact fees" that many jurisdictions levy on new housing rarely make up for the expenses of development. Taxpayers and utility rate payers, regardless of where they live, pay the remaining costs. Simply requiring new development to pay its own way, rather than being subsidized by taxpayers, would foster compact neighborhoods and infill development, where infrastructure costs are lower.

In the same vein, vehicle-related fees—fuel taxes, license and registration fees, and the like—cover only part of the costs of roads, bridges, public parking spaces, and other public expenses of driving. Taxpayers, even those who drive little, pick up the rest of the tab. If drivers had to pay the full costs for owning and operating their automobiles, they would pay more to drive—and, as a consequence, they would be less inclined to choose places to live where destinations are far apart and where driving is a necessity for every trip.

These three steps are just a starting point; other examples of public policies that could reduce automobile dependence and promote healthier land-use patterns can be found in previous volumes from Sightline Institute.

Unlike Snow's pump-handle solution, the steps we take now to curb sprawl will not take effect overnight. It may take years or even decades for the full benefits of these innovations to materialize. But just as Cascadians radically transformed their urban landscapes in the decades following World War II, they will rebuild much of what now exists over the coming half century. The question is what they will build. If they choose well, they will create cities with vital economies, safe and secure neighborhoods, flourishing communities, and low and diminishing environmental impacts. They will create cities where—with almost no one noticing at first—threats from car crashes will abate and opportunities to walk safely will abound. If northwesterners choose well, they will end up with a human habitat worthy of its creators. And they will set an example for the world.

ACKNOWLEDGMENTS

This edition of the Cascadia Scorecard is dedicated to David V. Yaden, in appreciation of his long and dedicated service as board chair of Sightline Institute from 1999 to 2005. With his deep wisdom and steady hand, Dave has steered Sightline through many narrow passages.

Cascadia Scorecard 2006: Focus on Sprawl & Health was written by Sightline staff Clark Williams-Derry, Eric de Place, and Alan Thein Durning, with research assistance from research consultant and intern Jessica Branom-Zwick. We thank others who helped with research and provided critical data, including CommEn Space staff Matt Stevenson and Chris Davis, who created most of the wildlife maps and the traffic fatalities map presented in the book; Josh Livni, who created the walkability maps of King County; Andrea Laliberte of the US Department of Agriculture, who provided GIS data on our wildlife range maps; and Lawrence Frank, Jim Chapman, and Sarah Kavage of Lawrence Frank and Company, Inc., who provided GIS data and guidance on the relationship between sprawl and walking in King County neighborhoods, and sprawl and health generally. We also thank book designer Jennifer Shontz, editor Julie Van Pelt, and proofreader Sherri Schultz.

We are grateful to our many volunteers for their valuable contributions in 2005, including communications interns Elizabeth Burton, Josh Finn, Melissa Mueller, and Peter White; development interns Erin Frost and Kevan Lee; and many other volunteers who donated time and skills, including Jessica Alan, Bonnie Amdur, Will Anderson, Mieke Bomann, Devon Bushnell, Elizabeth Cuneo, Rebecca Dougherty, J. D. Estes, William Feinberg, Laura Fisher, Carrie Fox, Geoff Grosenbach, Sonja Gustafson, Daniel Hornal, Nancy Johnson, Mark Kotzer, Andrew

Martin, Ashley Mitchell, George Murray, Sonya Noor, Todd Panek, Len Pavelka, Laurie Rechholtz, Roddy Scheer, Matt Schoellhamer, Owen Smith, Ahren Stroming, and Joeve and Porter Wilkinson. Particular thanks goes to two website volunteers, graphic designer Laura Bentley and search-and-replace whiz David Boctor; and to web developer extraordinaire Andrew Burkhalter, for bringing sightline.org to life. We also give special thanks to longtime Boise volunteer Lyn McCollum, who has kept us up to date on relevant news for 12 years.

We thank partners and experts who peer-reviewed Sightline's work and assisted with outreach in 2005, including Lisa Andrews, Dori Gilels, K. C. Golden, John Harrison, Cylvia Hayes, Patrick Mazza, MaryAnn O'Hara, Kim Radtke, Jessyn Schor, Joshua Skov, Eric Sorensen, Joe Thwaites, Heather Weiner, and the staff of Washington Toxics Coalition; as well as Laura Gerber and Andrea Riseden-Perry, two mothers who participated in our study of PBDEs. We also thank Christian Hagen at the Oregon Department of Fish and Wildlife and Wayne Wakkinen at the Idaho Department of Fish and Game for providing data for the book; and volunteer blog authors Yoram Bauman, Rich Feldman, Jen Lamson, Hans Peter Meyer, Thomas Michael Power, Dan Staley, Tim Steury, and Seth Zuckerman.

In 2005, Sightline benefited from the generosity of those who hosted, organized, or headlined events or discussion groups on our behalf, including Gail Achterman; John and Jane Emrick; Christine Hanna and Eugene Pitcher; Jeanette Henderson; Molly Keating and Glenn Rodriguez; Alex Loeb and Ethan Meginnes; Mithun; Sara Moorehead and Jeffrey Ratté; Ingrid Rasch; Laura Retzler and Henry Wigglesworth; Lura Smith and Bill Shubach; and David and Janice Yaden. And we are especially grateful to educator and performance artist Peter Donaldson, who performed his Leonardo da Vinci show at two Sightline benefits.

Sightline thanks its board of directors for their donation of much time and support: board chair John Atcheson, and board members Gail Achterman, Alan Thein Durning, Jeff Hallberg, Ethan Meginnes, Gordon

Price, Allen Puckett, Laura Retzler, and David Yaden. We would also like to thank former board members who completed their service in 2005, including Catherine Mater, Nancy Olewiler, and Aron Thompson.

Finally, Sightline is grateful to its hardworking staff: senior research associate Eric de Place, development director Peter Drury, executive director Alan Thein Durning, managing director Christine Hanna, Tidepool editor Kristin Kolb-Angelbeck, communications director Elisa Murray, grants associate Madeline Ostrander, senior development associate Stacey Panek, senior communications associate Leigh Sims, and research director Clark Williams-Derry. We also thank former staff Dana Brown (operations manager/bookkeeper) and Parke Burgess (director of donor relations), and Jessica Branom-Zwick (research intern and research consultant).

OUR SUPPORTERS

GIFTS & COMMITMENTS FOR 2005

The gifts and commitments listed below were received from January 1 through December 31, 2005. We would like to thank these donors, together with all who supported our mission in 2005. We wish to express particular appreciation for the Cascadia Stewards Council, comprising those who have made multiyear financial commitments at a level of $1,000 annually or greater to help fuel the work of Sightline. Members of the Cascadia Stewards Council are listed in boldface type, and an asterisk (*) denotes a Founding Member of the Council.

$100,000 or more
The Russell Family Foundation

$25,000–$99,999
Contorer Foundation*
The Glaser Progress Foundation
Social Venture Partners

$10,000–$24,999
Aveda Corporation
The Brainerd Foundation
Tom & Sonya Campion*
Horizons Foundation
Anonymous*
Microsoft (Matching Gifts Program)
Linda S. Park & Denis G. Janky*
Seattle Biotech Legacy Foundation
The Seattle Foundation

$5,000–$9,999
Jabe Blumenthal & Julie Edsforth*
Harvey Jones & Nancy Iannucci
Jubitz Family Foundation
Loeb/Meginnes Foundation*
Judy Pigott*
Laura Retzler & Henry Wigglesworth*
Christopher & Mary Troth*
Doug & Maggie Walker (Walker Family Foundation)

$2,500–4,999
John Atcheson*
Magali & Jeffrey Belt*
David Callahan
Mary A. Crocker Trust for Elizabeth Atcheson
Gun & Tom Denhart*
Anonymous
Alan & Amy Thein Durning*
Richard & Sara Farmer
The Hugh & Jane Ferguson Foundation
Robert & Judy Fisher
Maggie Hooks & Justin Ferrari*
The Mountaineers Foundation
John Russell & Mary Fellows*
Janet Vogelzang & Mark Cliggett*

$1,001–2,499
Gail L. Achterman*
Amgen Foundation (Matching Gifts Program)
Erin & Jonathan Becker
Brian & Sharon Beinlich
Parke G. Burgess Jr*
Jon Carder & Monique Baillargeon*
Peter Donaldson*
Jonathan Durning & Melanie Ronai*
Environmental Support Center
Lowell & Nancy Ericsson
Maradel Krummel Gale*

Hellmut & Marcy Golde
Mark Groudine & Cynthia Putnam*
Christine Hanna & Eugene Pitcher*
Harris Bank Foundation
Jeanette L. Henderson*
George Hess
Kristayani & Jerry Jones (The Oregon Community Foundation)*
Mark A. Kotzer & Lauren Adler*
David Lahaie & Petra Franklin Lahaie
Tom & Jennifer Luce*
Langdon Marsh & Ellie Putnam*
Karen & Jeremy Mazner*
Edward Mills & Irene Pasternack*
The Mitzvah Foundation
James L. Plummer*
Glenn S. Rodriguez & Molly E. R. Keating*
Carrie & Barry Saxifrage
Washington Mutual (Matching Gifts Program)
Janice & David Yaden*
Jeff Youngstrom & Becky Brooks*

$1,000
David Ahlers & Liza Sheehan
J. F. & Leslie Baken*
Paul & Donna Balle*
Connie Battaile*
Gordon Battaile
The Estate of Julian Battaile*
Tony & Sue Beeman*
Anonymous*
Anonymous
Thomas Buxton & Terri Anderson*
Ann & Doug Christensen*
Grace K. Dinsdale*
Jean & Marvin Durning
John & Jane Emrick*
Nigel Green & Lisa Chin
Jeff & Nicole Hallberg*

Anonymous*
Erik & Gretchen Jansen*
Keith Kegley*
Bill Kramer & Melissa Cadwallader*
Matt & Leslie Leber (Seattle Pacific Gift Fund)
Anonymous
Mithun
Sara Moorehead & Jeffrey Ratté*
Linda Moulder & Jerry White*
Tanya & Patrick Niemeyer
The Pfizer Foundation (Matching Gifts Program)
Jean Marie Piserchia & Robert C. Ball*
James & Rebecca Potter*
Gordon Price & Len Sobo*
Allen & Laura Puckett
Ingrid Rasch*
Mike & Faye Richardson
Doane Rising
Jo Roberts
Abbe Sue Rubin
Anirudh Sahni*
Manya & Howard Shapiro*
Sonya M. Stoklosa (Mellon Private Wealth Management)
Valerie Tarico & Brian Arbogast
Jim & Jan Thomas*
Birgitte B. Williams*
Winky Foundation

$250–$999
Victoria Burwell
Vincent Celie & Aileen Murphy
Mary Anne Christy & Mark Klebanoff
David & Wendy Cohan
Curtis DeGasperi & Sara Waterman
William Feinberg
Albert E. Foster
Diana Gale & Jerome Hillis
Bill & Melinda Gates Foundation

Richard Gibson & Carol Peterkort
WM Ross Gillanders & Eregina Bradford
Michel Girard
Wendy Green
William & Barbara Harris
Sara Stewart Hinckley
Lisa Hoffman & Bill Driscoll
Vincent Houmes
David Huffaker & Barbara Staley
Livia Jackson
Lars & Eva B. Johansson
Eugene Kahn
Neil Kelly, Inc.
Frances & David Korten
The Arie Kurtzig Memorial Fund
Nancy-Clair Laird & Steven McInaney
Clemens J. Laufenberg
The Lawrence Family Fund (The Oregon
    Community Foundation)
Robert B. Loken
John & Hanna Liv Mahlum Trust
Richard Meyer & Aleta Howard
Tom & Sue Millan (Millan Family Trust)
Deborah & John Munson
Jennifer Myhre & Mike Jerome
Ann Parker-Way & Paul Way
Leonard E. Pavelka
Katherine A. Randolph & Kyle Wang
Laurie Rechholtz
Peter W. Riggs
Carol D. Roberts
Ross & Associates Environmental Consulting, Ltd.
Scott & C. Joan Sandberg
John & Lorrie Schleg
Peter & Rita Thein
Kristopher & Jo Ann Townsend
Kathryn E. Wilbur
Pete & Joeve Wilkinson
Kenneth G. & Yvonne M. Zick

IN-KIND DONATIONS

We are grateful to the following individuals and organizations who donated valuable services or material gifts to Sightline in 2005.

Anonymous
Gail Achterman
Peter Alsop
Steven Cristol
DLA Piper Rudnick Gray Cary US LLC
Peter Donaldson
Gordon Dow
Alan & Amy Thein Durning
egg Advertising
John & Jane Emrick
Christine Hanna & Eugene Pitcher
Heckler Associates
Jeanette L. Henderson
Lexicon Branding
Alex Loeb & Ethan Meginnes
Mithun
Sara Moorehead & Jeffrey Ratté
Nonprofit Recruitment Services
Judy Pigott
Ingrid Rasch
Laura Retzler & Henry Wigglesworth
Glenn S. Rodriguez & Molly E. R. Keating
Lura Smith & Bill Shubach
Social Venture Partners
Glenn Thomas
Weiss Jenkins Properties
David & Janice Yaden